PENGUIN BOOKS

LIVING EASY WITH DIABETES

Dr Pradeep G. Talwalkar has been practising diabetology for three decades now. Formerly a postgraduate teacher of internal medicine, he now teaches diabetology.

A sought-after speaker at various conferences, symposiums and continuing medical education programmes, Dr Talwalkar has lectured extensively all over India. He is very active on the patient education front: besides conducting workshops and seminars, he uses the print, radio, television and online media to spread awareness about diabetes among patients and caregivers.

Dr Talwalkar has attended numerous international conferences on diabetes and visited several centres of excellence in the field. He has actively participated in all conferences of the International Diabetes Federation since the 1988 conference in Sydney, Australia. He has authored over fifty papers in national and international journals, and written and edited books on diabetes for laypeople, family physicians and consultants. He is the assistant editor of *API Textbook of Medicine* (sixth edition), a popular textbook with wide readership in India.

Living Easy with
Diabetes
The *Ultimate* Handbook

DR PRADEEP G. TALWALKAR

PENGUIN BOOKS

An imprint of Penguin Random House

PENGUIN BOOKS

USA | Canada | UK | Ireland | Australia
New Zealand | India | South Africa | China | Singapore

Penguin Books is part of the Penguin Random House group of companies
whose addresses can be found at global.penguinrandomhouse.com

Published by Penguin Random House India Pvt. Ltd
4th Floor, Capital Tower 1, MG Road,
Gurugram 122 002, Haryana, India

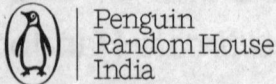

Penguin
Random House
India

First published by Penguin Books India 2013

ISBN 9780143419723

Typeset in Sabon by R. Ajith Kumar, New Delhi
Printed at Repro India Limited

www.penguin.co.in

I am deeply indebted to my patients for
listening to me and giving me the opportunity
to hone my skills in patient education.
I dedicate this book to all my patients.

CONTENTS

Appendices

INTRODUCTION

I have been practising as a diabetologist for about three decades. Early in my career, I realized that many of my patients with diabetes—and these included those that had been diabetic for a long time as well as those who were highly educated—were not at all knowledgeable about or clued-up on the nitty-gritty of diabetes. In other words, they were 'diabetes illiterate'. Moreover, they had numerous misconceptions about diabetes. This, in my opinion, is a major obstacle on the path to achieving persistently good blood glucose control and thus preventing or significantly postponing the dreaded complications of diabetes and leading a healthy and high quality life.

I sincerely believe that a 'diabetes illiterate' patient reflects poorly on the ability of his treating physician. Educating and sensitizing the patient is an integral part of the overall management of diabetes. If a patient does not understand the importance of constant monitoring and regular treatment, he will never totally comply with the doctor's advice and, as a result, will struggle to achieve blood glucose control.

There has been tremendous activity in the field of diabetes research and management in the last few years. And yet there is no sign of a decline in the epidemic of diabetes. As per a study by the Indian Council of Medical Research (ICMR), published in the October 2011 issue of *Diabetologia*, India has 62.4 million diabetic patients and 77.2 million pre-diabetics (a condition preceding diabetes, in which blood glucose levels are higher than normal, though not in the diabetes range). As per earlier projections made by the International Diabetes Federation (IDF) in 2009, India was likely to have 47 million diabetics by 2010 and 79 million diabetics by 2030. However, on the basis of the ICMR study, India is likely to have about 100 million diabetics by 2030. The diagnostic criterion for diabetes for fasting blood glucose value has been lowered from 140 mg%[1] to 126 mg% because some patients have been diagnosed with diabetic retinopathy (an eye complication specific to diabetes) at blood glucose levels lower than 140 mg%. In fact, the lowest fasting blood glucose level at which diabetic retinopathy has been documented is 126 mg%. The higher limit for normal fasting blood glucose has also been reduced from 110 mg% to 100 mg%.

There have been some changes in the classification of diabetes as well. The science of diabetology has evolved (not at the rate we would have liked it to, though) and we now know more about diabetes than ever before. In the last few years, several new anti-diabetic pills and injections have been introduced in India. Diabetics and those interested to know more about it would naturally like to keep pace with these new developments. It is essential for a diabetic to acquire

---

1   mg% is a unit to express the level of glucose concentration in the blood. It implies milligrams per 100 ml or milligrams per decilitre (mg/dl).

working knowledge of various aspects of diabetes. Knowledge is one of the four pillars on which successful management of diabetes rests. This has motivated me to write this simple yet comprehensive book for patients with diabetes and pre-diabetes and others, such as caregivers, who want to learn more about it.

Living Easy with Diabetes is essentially a handbook, written in simple and easy language, with the sincere aim of educating diabetics and their close relatives and friends who are involved in caring for them on a daily basis. The idea is to provide the readers with important information on various aspects of diabetes—information that should be complementary to the medical advice provided by the treating physician or diabetologist. Diabetes is a lifelong disease and therefore requires lifelong commitment from diabetics.

Diabetes is also a silent disease. Typical symptoms of diabetes develop only after a patient's blood glucose shoots up to a very high level, say greater than 400 mg%. (Please note that the acceptable blood glucose levels are 70 mg%–130 mg% for pre-meal blood glucose and under 180 mg% for post-meal blood glucose, as benchmarked by the American Diabetes Association.) Even mildly elevated blood glucose levels over long periods, a few months or years, are sufficient to cause significant damage to vital organs such as eyes, kidneys and heart. The danger is that during this phase of mild blood glucose elevation, patients do not exhibit any classic symptoms of diabetes and falsely believe that they must be doing well on the diabetes front. Pressing needs of day-to-day life take priority over medical check-ups. It is important to understand that no matter how good he or she feels, a diabetic must go for regular, periodic check-ups.

Consider the real-life case of forty-five-year-old Anand, an ambitious and hard-working businessman. Last year, Anand was deeply involved in the construction of a new factory to meet the growing market demand for his products. For six months, he almost forgot about his diabetes and neglected his exercise, diet and medication regimen. When his neighbour was diagnosed with gangrene brought on by uncontrolled diabetes, he remembered that he too was a diabetic and resolved to be sincere in following his diet, exercise and medication. He quickly underwent investigations to ensure that he was still free from complications of diabetes despite inadequate control over his blood glucose over the preceding six months. He thanked god that he had indeed escaped the complications, remembering another incident from two years ago when he had escaped unscathed from a high-speed car accident on the busy Mumbai–Pune expressway. Anand never forgets these two incidents, and thanks god profusely for letting him escape unharmed both times.

While he did get away unscarred from the car episode, has he really come away unblemished from the six-month period of uncontrolled diabetes? No complications were detected at the end of that period but is Anand unaffected? The answer is NO. The negative effects of uncontrolled diabetes are not felt or detected in a relatively short period but each day of uncontrolled diabetes compounds the problems and, when it reaches a threshold, complications develop.

Anand has fully understood now that the two incidents are far from similar. If he wants to live a long, quality life free of diabetes-related handicaps, he has to keep his blood glucose under control 24/7, every day of his life. In fact, he now considers persistent and strict blood glucose control as an intangible investment in the long-term success of his business.

Through this book, I hope to motivate diabetics and pre-diabetics to take control of their lives and their condition by providing them vital information on diabetes including the advantages of prudent monitoring and management, and also by reassuring them that there is no need to despair if one is disciplined and methodical. A diabetic can lead a normal or near-normal life if he is careful about all aspects of diabetes management including diet, exercise and medication. The book deals with the practical aspects of diabetes—how to administer insulin injections; travel tips; marriage and sexual relations; employment issues—as well as common misunderstandings and tips on preventing diabetes. Diabetes can be prevented or considerably postponed by early identification of pre-diabetes, and subsequently by implementing prudent exercise and dietary programmes in those who have pre-diabetes.

The pioneering American diabetologist Dr Elliott Proctor Joslin said, 'The diabetic who knows the most will live the longest.' I hope that my readers will be motivated into persistent and prudent management of diabetes and thus succeed in leading a normal life despite having diabetes.

Should you have any queries after reading this book, do write to me at pg_talwalkar@hotmail.com and I will personally address your queries.

1

WHAT IS DIABETES?

In verbal as well as written communication, the word 'diabetes' is used as a short form for the condition called diabetes mellitus (DM). Do note, however, that there is another extremely rare type of diabetes called diabetes incipidus (DI). Excessive urination and thirst are common symptoms in those with uncontrolled DM and DI. However, those with DI do not face insulin deficiency, so their blood glucose (sugar) is always within normal range.

The diabetic condition or *madhumeha* was first described in writing in 1500 BCE in Indian Ayurvedic texts that documented how flies and ants were attracted to the urine of people with a mysterious disease that caused intense thirst, enormous urine output and wasting away of the body. The word diabetes was first used in 230 BCE by Apollonius of Egypt, who derived it from the Greek word for 'siphon' or 'to go through', implying that the disease drained more fluid than a person could consume. Then, in the late seventeenth century, the British doctor Thomas Willis added the term *mellitus*, the Latin word for 'honeyed', because the condition made urine sweet.

In this book, the word diabetes is used to denote DM, which includes a group of disorders in which there is absolute or relative deficiency of insulin, a hormone produced by the pancreas, an endocrine gland situated in the upper abdomen behind the stomach.

Insulin, an important anabolic (constructive or bodybuilding) hormone, has a profound effect on human metabolism, including carbohydrate metabolism. More than 60 per cent of the calories in our food comes from carbohydrates, which are converted into glucose or simple sugars at the end of the process of digestion. This glucose leaves the intestine to enter the bloodstream and then circulates to all the tissues and cells of the body. It is insulin that helps glucose enter cells, particularly in the muscles, where some of it is broken down to provide instant energy and the rest is stored in the form of glycogen (a complex sugar) for use later when the body needs a sudden spurt of energy, say, during a state of fasting. Insulin also prevents the formation of glucose in the liver. Through this two-pronged action—(1) facilitating the movement of glucose from the blood into the tissues and (2) regulating the formation of glucose in the liver—insulin helps to maintain blood glucose concentration within a normal range.

What happens in the diabetic condition is that either insulin is not produced at all (as in type 1 DM) or there is an insulin deficiency, either actual or relative (as in type 2 DM). The latter is the commonest type of DM, covering about 96 per cent of diabetics in India.

Diabetes is a condition in which there is absolute or relative deficiency of insulin, a hormone produced by the beta cells in the pancreas, an endocrine gland. The deficiency of insulin leads to a rise in blood glucose levels.

In type 2 DM, insulin production is very erratic. The pancreas produces varying amounts of insulin. In some cases, particularly in the initial periods, pre-diabetics as well as diabetics produce even more insulin than non-diabetics do. However, the tissues of diabetics are less sensitive to insulin than those of non-diabetics; they require more insulin than normal to keep their blood glucose levels in the normal range. In the initial period, before the onset of diabetes as well as in the initial years of the condition, the pancreas produces and releases more insulin to compensate for the reduced tissue sensitivity. As the insulin resistance persists and insulin demand increases, a time comes when the beta cells[1] in the pancreas fail to keep up the supply. At this stage, these people develop relative insulin deficiency and that leads to diabetes.

---

1 Beta cells are situated in the islets of Langerhans, islands of hormone-producing cells in the pancreas. In normal conditions, these cells constantly assess the prevailing blood glucose level and accordingly alter the rate of insulin production and release. When blood glucose rises, for instance after a meal, they release more insulin into the bloodstream. When blood glucose falls, as in a fasting state, they temporarily suspend insulin release.

Insulin controls blood glucose by:

⬆ Facilitating entry of glucose in tissues
&
⬇ Inhibiting formation of glucose in the liver

In diabetes there is insulin deficiency,
thus

⬇ Glucose uptake by the tissues is reduced
&
⬆ Glucose production in the liver is increased
thus
⬆ blood glucose rises

Obesity is associated with reduced sensitivity or resistance to insulin. Many obese people overcome this impairment simply by producing more insulin to maintain normal blood glucose levels. However, those obese people who have inherited beta cell defects are unable to cope with the gradually increasing demand made by their tissues for more and more insulin. As a fallout of this demand–supply mismatch, they develop diabetes. This would explain why obesity is commonly associated with diabetes. However, obese people without beta cell defects—whether inherited or acquired—have unlimited capacity to produce insulin as per demand and so they do not develop diabetes even though they are obese and have insulin resistance. If you consider the corollary, you will realize that it is not necessary for a person to be obese to develop diabetes. People with absolutely normal body weight too can turn diabetic if they have severe beta cell defects. In India, in fact, the relationship between general obesity and diabetes is not as pronounced as in the western countries.

Remember, every obese person is not diabetic and every diabetic need not be obese.

2

HOW WIDESPREAD IS DIABETES?

The sheer rise in the incidence of diabetes across the world, and right here in India, is significant and disturbing. Of the 360 million diabetics in the world today, 62.4 million are in India, making it home to the world's second largest diabetic population, after China with 92 million diabetics. What is more, the prevalence of diabetes or the percentage of population suffering from diabetes is rapidly on the rise in India. According to a survey carried out by the Indian Council of Medical Research (ICMR), in 1971, 1.5 per cent of rural adults and 2.3 per cent of urban adults in India had diabetes. In the decade 2000–2010, these figures shot up to 4.26 per cent and 12.1 per cent, respectively.[1] By 2030, when the global diabetic population will increst to 439 million, India alone will have a whopping 100 million diabetics.

> Every eight seconds, across the world, two people are diagnosed as having diabetes. Every eight seconds, somewhere in the world, one diabetic dies.

1 A. Ramchandran, 'Pandemic of Diabetes in India and Potential Solutions', in *Innovative Approaches to Type 2 Diabetes*, edited by Jayram B.M (Micro Labs: Bangalore 2012), pp. 1–8.

Why is diabetes on the rise? Here are some reasons:

- *More mechanization, less physical exercise:* Our forefathers used their legs to walk and climb, or their hands to mix and grind—we use cars and elevators, and food processors.

- *Forgotten traditional foods, newer junk foods:* We consume a lot of 'energy-dense' fast food instead of traditional, freshly cooked food rich in roughage. Ready-to-eat foods often contain refined cereals instead of whole grains; for instance, bread, pizza and pasta are usually made from maida instead of wheat flour like chapattis. Salads and green leafy vegetables are rich in unabsorbable fibres and they provide a smaller amount of calories per volume of food as compared with ready-made dishes (made with refined flours), which are poorer in unabsorbable fibres and richer in oils and fats, thus yielding more calories per food volume and being labelled energy-dense.

- *Phasing out the rural, ushering in the urban:* Our population is migrating very rapidly from a slow-paced rural milieu to a much faster-paced cosmopolitan lifestyle. Exposure to this alien, aggressive, competitive atmosphere creates tremendous stress. Let me quote the noted epidemiologist, Dr Paul Zimmet, 'Industrialization and Coca-colonization have ruined civilization.'

- *Decline of diseases, advent of longevity:* DM is essentially a disease of middle age and beyond. At the time of India's Independence in 1947, the average life expectancy of Indians was about forty years. Significant economic and scientific progress made since Independence have led to a sharp fall in mortality from nutritional deficiencies and germ-linked diseases, thus ushering in longevity. The life expectancy of Indians today is sixty years. This means that more Indians now survive to develop diabetes. Moreover, with better diagnostic facilities even in non-urban areas, the condition of diabetes is now diagnosed clearly and in a larger number of people.

For quite some time now, the prevalence of diabetes in Indians settled abroad has been much higher than in the local populations. Surveys conducted in the UK, the US, the Fiji Islands and Mauritius have confirmed this.[2] Until the 1990s, we were under the false belief that the prevalence of diabetes in native Indians is much lower. We now know that, at least in urban India, the prevalence of diabetes is very high. By the end of the 2030s, India will have over 100 million diabetics.

As per the ICMR-INDIAB 2011 study[3] (see graphs on the facing page) in Tamil Nadu, Maharashtra, Jharkhand and Chandigarh, and extrapolated to derive all-India figures, India already has 62.4 million diabetics and is likely to surpass IDF's figure of 79.4 million much before 2030. The following graphs depict the increasing prevalence of diabetes and pre-diabetes in India.

---

2 P.Z. Zimmet, 'Challenges in Diabetes Epidemiology from West to the Rest', *Diabetes Care* 2: 232–52.

3 ICMR-INDIAB (Indian Council of Medical Research and India Diabetes Study collaborative group), 'Prevalence of diabetes and pre-diabetes in urban and rural India (Phase 1 results)', *Diabetologia* 293: 217–28.

There is a large variation in the prevalence of type 2 DM across communities. The highest rates are found in

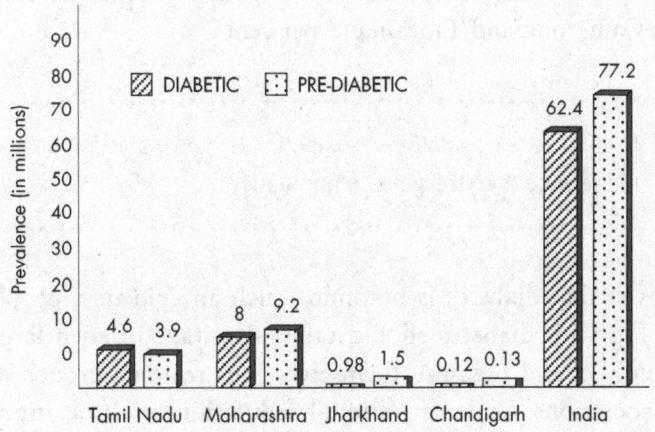

HIGH PREVALENCE OF DIABETES IN INDIA: 2011
SOURCE: ICMR-INDIAB 2011

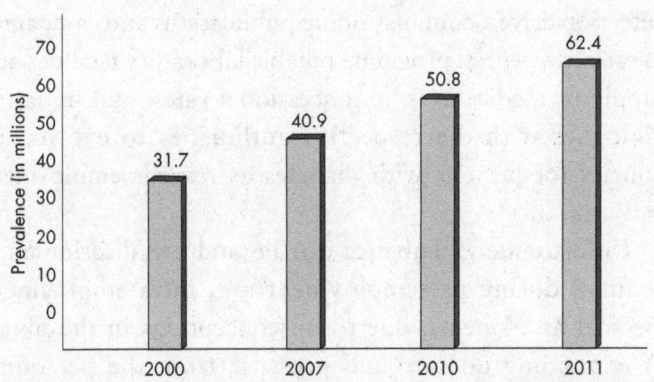

INCREASING PREVALENCE OF DIABETES IN INDIA: 2011
SOURCE: ICMR-INDIAB 2011

some native American tribes such as Pima Indians (over 50 per cent) while low prevalence rates are found in the least developed rural communities in many African countries, such as Cameroon and Tanzania (3 per cent).

In India, the population of diabetics is growing at a much higher rate than the general population!

Given that diabetes is becoming such an epidemic, people living with diabetes should take advantage of such large numbers and organize themselves into regional groups or associations, under a national federation of associations perhaps. Such robust and organized associations would help improve the quality of life of diabetics in various ways: organizing informative lectures, group discussions, and detection drives; commissioning publications and campaigns to raise awareness; providing reliable laboratory facilities and supply of medications at concessional rates; and initiating dialogues with the respective authorities to evolve fair policies for persons with diabetes as regards employment and insurance.

Unfortunately, diabetics can be and are discriminated against, during pre-employment and intra-employment medical assessments, due to misconceptions in the minds of examining doctors and pressure from the personnel departments of employers. Let me give you a classic example— even senior medical consultants can be misinformed!

A driver from a car pool of the Maharashtra government exhibiting a marginally high blood glucose level was referred to me for a fitness certificate. His job was to escort visiting dignitaries from Mumbai airport into the city. Since most of the time he had nothing to do but sit and wait patiently, he had become overweight, with a mildly elevated blood glucose level. He did not have any complications and all he needed to do was reduce his weight by exercising regularly and controlling his diet. Since he did not require medicines to bring down his blood glucose, he was unlikely to get sudden hypoglycaemia (a state of low blood sugar discussed in Chapter 12), which could be dangerous, particularly while driving. During a severe hypoglycaemic episode, the patient gets confused and is unable to take quick decisions or make judgement calls.

I had no hesitation in declaring him fit for his job, but with the remark that he should get his blood glucose tested regularly and go for medical checks to assess organ functions and detect any complications related to diabetes. A very senior doctor who was present while I assessed this driver remarked that he would never certify him fit for driving. I find this very unfair. One has to individualize decisions considering the type and severity of diabetes, the type of job and the presence or absence of complications such as impaired vision, high blood pressure and heart disease.

Why Should I Control Diabetes?

Diseases of the large blood vessels are commonly associated with diabetes, due to accelerated hardening and narrowing of major arteries. If the blood vessels of the brain are affected, the result can be a paralytic stroke. If the blood vessels of the heart are afflicted, the patient can have a heart attack and heart failure. If the major blood vessels of the leg are narrowed, the diabetic can end up developing gangrene and may have to lose the affected leg. These processes can be slowed down considerably if one controls diabetes prudently and persistently.

It has indeed been proven beyond doubt that troublesome complications of diabetes such as retinopathy leading to blindness, kidney disease leading to the need for dialysis or transplantation for survival, and gangrene of the feet and legs leading to amputation can be prevented or considerably postponed if blood glucose is controlled persistently and painstakingly. These complications are specific to diabetes and are responsible for considerable morbidity (handicaps such as blindness, loss of leg, etc.) and mortality (loss of life).

Persistent rise in blood glucose damages the capillary endothelium (inner lining of small blood vessels), which causes blood to leak out from the capillaries into the surrounding tissues and damage them. When small blood vessels in the retina get damaged (diabetic retinopathy), it can ultimately lead to blindness; it is, in fact, the commonest cause of blindness in the developed world as well as among financially better-off patients in India. The affection of capillaries in the kidneys (diabetic nephropathy) ultimately leads to end-stage kidney failure, necessitating either a kidney transplant or dialysis three times a week for one's entire lifetime, both extremely expensive procedures and beyond the reach of many.

Diabetic neuropathy or nerve damage causes unbearable pain and numbness in the legs, and this interferes with daily activities and sleep, thus totally incapacitating the patient. Impaired sensation in the legs is one of the major factors responsible for 'diabetic foot' lesions, which can lead to gangrene and result in foot/leg amputation.

Long-standing diabetes can lead to nerve damage or diabetic neuropathy and can result in organic impotence, thus affecting your sexual health and conjugal relationships.

If blood glucose is kept under control persistently, one can also prevent infections such as tuberculosis, pneumonia, skin and soft tissue infections and fungal infections, which can cause morbidity. Moreover, in emergent situations, morbidity and mortality are definitely lower in diabetics whose blood glucose is well controlled.

To reiterate, the only way to prevent all these complications is to meticulously and relentlessly manage diabetes.

Till the mid-1990s, there was no concrete proof (based on properly designed long-term clinical research) about the beneficial effects of strict blood glucose control. The scenario has transformed since the publication of the results of the Diabetes Control and Complication Trial (DCCT) undertaken by the National Institute of Diabetes and Digestive and Kidney Diseases (US) from 1983 through 1993. This monumental research work, done in the US and Canada on type 1 diabetics, assessed the effect of intensive versus conventional insulin therapy on diabetic complications like retinopathy, nephropathy and neuropathy in 1441 patients over six and a half years.

Intensive therapy meant at least three insulin injections daily, at least four self-examinations of blood glucose daily with a glucometer and frequent feedback to the investigators. Conventional therapy meant one to two insulin injections daily, one self-examination of blood glucose daily and less frequent communication with the investigators. At the end of the trial, it was found that type 1 diabetics on intensive treatment had a 50 per cent reduced risk of developing retinopathy, nephropathy and neuropathy, and of progression of micro-vascular lesions as compared with those on conventional treatment.

The Diabetes Control and Complication Trial by the National Institute of Diabetes and Digestive and Kidney Diseases (US) showed that keeping blood sugar levels as close to normal as possible slows the onset and progression of eye, kidney and nerve damage caused by diabetes. In fact, it demonstrated that any sustained lowering of blood sugar helps, even if the person has a history of poor control.

Read more at http://diabetes.niddk.nih.gov/dm/pubs/control/

After this major milestone in diabetes research came the United Kingdom Prospective Diabetes Study (UKPDS) in 1997, the biggest clinical trial ever undertaken in the field of diabetes till then, this time with type 2 diabetics. It proved that better blood glucose control through intensive management of diabetes can lead to significant reductions in complications as compared with conventional treatment. More than 5000 newly diagnosed type 2 diabetics participated and were followed up for an average of seven years. In a side study, it was also proven that in those diabetics who also had high blood pressure, intensive treatment with blood pressure medications significantly reduced mortality and morbidity compared with conventional treatment for blood pressure.

The Steno 2 study[4] was a small but very elaborate study done on 160 patients in the Netherlands. Outcomes of aggressive multi-factorial interventions with medicines to control blood glucose, blood pressure, cholesterol and platelet clogging with aspirin were compared with conventional and conservative treatment over a period of nearly eight years. Patients in the aggressive arm of the trial enjoyed a 58 per cent reduction in cardiovascular problems. Subsequently, patients in both the groups were asked to choose their treatment (aggressive or conservative) for a further period of five and a half years. At the end of this period, despite deterioration in blood glucose, blood pressure and cholesterol control due to their having chosen the less aggressive approach, the patients who were earlier in the aggressive arm continued to be protected from cardiovascular problems.

---

4 Peter Gæde, Pernille Vedel, Nicolai Larsen, Gunnar V.H. Jensen, Hans-Henrik Parving, and Oluf Pedersen, 'Multi-factorial Interventions and Cardiovascular Disease in Patients with Type 2 Diabetes', *New England Journal of Medicine* 348: 383–93.

Metabolic Memory (Legacy Effect)

In the last fifteen years, there have been several comprehensive and well-designed long-term research studies (DCCT, UKPDS, Steno 2, etc.) comparing aggressive and conventional management of blood glucose, blood pressure and lipids.

In the DCCT, aggressive insulin therapy was compared with conventional insulin therapy. In the main UKPDS, aggressive therapy for blood glucose control was compared with conventional therapy. In the Steno 2 study, simultaneous aggressive management of high blood glucose, high blood pressure and high lipids was compared with conventional management of the same factors.

As expected, aggressively managed patients in both the DCCT and the UKPDS had better blood glucose control and fewer complications at the end of the study period. Similarly, aggressively treated patients in the Steno 2 study had better control of blood glucose, blood pressure and lipids, and thus had fewer complications. At the end of these studies, the patients were given the option to continue the same treatment or cross over. Both groups were closely observed for another long-term period.

Over time, the differences in their values gradually reduced because most patients in the conventional arm of the original studies opted for aggressive treatment in the second phase while those who were originally in the aggressive arm yielded to some slackening in lifestyle as well as drug compliance. However, patients from the aggressive arm in the first phase still continued to benefit from the tighter controls and achievements of target values. Thus, at the end of the second phase, the difference in the rate of developing complications was maintained despite similar blood glucose control in the DCCT and UKPDS studies, while those who received aggressive management in the first phase of the Steno 2 study showed further reduced cardiovascular mortality.

The Hope study also threw up similar findings. This was a large study involving 9541 patients and ran for four and a half years in its first part. People with risk factors for cardiovascular disease or having type 2 diabetes were divided into two groups. One group was put on 10 mg of ramipril daily in addition to the routine diabetes, high blood pressure, high cholesterol and anti-platelet medications. The other group was given a placebo[5] in addition to all the other required medications.

In the group on ramipril, various complications like heart disease, kidney failure, paralytic stroke and diabetic retinopathy were significantly reduced. At the end of four and a half years, those on placebo were given the option of moving over to ramipril while those on ramipril were given the option of discontinuing. Most of those in the placebo group started on ramipril while some in the ramipril group discontinued it.

---

5 A placebo is a dummy pill that looks exactly like the active drug. It is used in research studies to evaluate the efficacy and safety of the drug under study. Patients are divided into two groups; one group is given the actual drug while the other group is given the placebo. The research is carried out in a 'double blind' manner—neither the patients nor the treating doctors are aware of who receives the active drug and who is on placebo. This eliminates any physician and patient bias while the results are evaluated.

At the end of the second phase, those originally on ramipril continued to benefit from its good effects and the gap between the relative rate of reduction of complications between the two groups widened. This phenomenon, where metabolic and vascular benefits are extended over years (despite some deterioration in control of blood glucose, blood pressure and lipids) in diabetics who earlier maintained persistent control over these parameters is known as the 'legacy effect' or 'metabolic memory effect'. Thus, those who detect their diabetes very early and succeed in controlling their blood glucose strictly in the initial years are richly rewarded for their efforts. What is the reward? Protection from diabetes-induced damage to vital organs even if blood glucose control is not as good as it should be in later years.

The implications of these studies are very important. Complications of diabetes can reduce life expectancy by five to ten years, reduce the quality of life and increase the cost of treatment exponentially. There is a strong case for early diagnosis of diabetes and immediate and aggressive management of blood glucose. All associated risk factors should be promptly identified and quickly brought under control. This will help our endeavour to prevent complications of diabetes and enable diabetics to live a long, quality life, just like those without diabetes.

THE CASE OF SOONER RATHER THAN LATER

Bharat and Ramesh are similar in many ways. Both are forty-one. Both have been diabetic for over a decade. Both comply religiously with medical advice on medication, diet and exercise. Both have good control over their blood glucose as indicated by their glycosylated haemoglobin values of 7 per cent and 6.9 per cent, respectively.

This is where the similarity ends. Bharat has no complications of diabetes but Ramesh has early kidney and eye complications. Why?

Ten years ago, Bharat's diabetes was diagnosed in a routine health check-up. He immediately went to an expert and meticulously followed his advice, maintaining tight control over his blood glucose all through the last decade. Ramesh waited for symptoms of diabetes such as thirst and excessive urination before going in for blood glucose tests, and was thus exposed to high blood glucose levels for a long time before he started treatment. Moreover, soon after he started treatment and felt better, he assumed that his blood glucose was well-controlled and he could relax his diet, exercise and medication plans. He often missed his scheduled blood tests. He was preoccupied with his career but, ironically, failed to understand the importance of investing in his health for his career. This resulted in poor blood glucose control in the crucial initial years after the diagnosis of diabetes. Four years ago, in a diabetes education programme, he realized his blunder. Subsequently, he has complied with his doctor's advice and managed tight blood glucose control for four years. But he missed the bus initially and now, despite good control, he has mild kidney and eye complications. It is still not too late, though. If he maintains persistent control from now on, he can significantly slow down deterioration in his kidney function and prevent visual impairment.

World Diabetic Population: An Interesting Break-Up

Number of diabetics in the world	360 million
Number of diabetics aware of their condition	180 million (50%)
Number of diabetics being treated	90 million (50% of known diabetics)
Number of diabetics at their blood glucose goals	45 million (50% of those being treated)
Number of diabetics with complications despite achieving blood glucose goals	22.5 million (50% of those at their blood sugar goals)

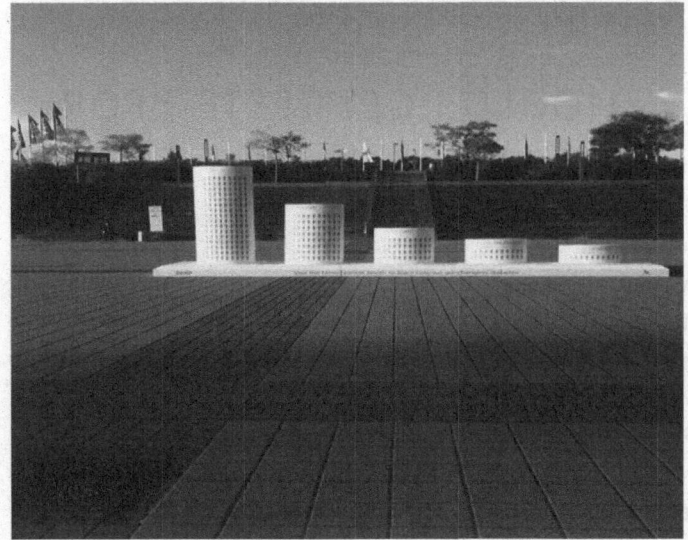

Photograph by Pradeep Talwalkar

This installation from the 2012 annual conference of the European Association for the Study of Diabetes (1–5 October 2012, Berlin) depicts the statistics in the chart given above through its five bars: first bar = 360 million, the number of diabetics in the world; second bar = 180 million, the number of diabetics aware of their condition; third bar = 90 million, the number of diabetics being treated; fourth bar = 45 million, the number of diabetics at their blood glucose goals; fifth bar = 22.5 million, the number of diabetics with complications despite reaching their blood glucose goals.

3

SHOULD I GET TESTED FOR DIABETES?

As you know now, diabetes can creep into your system and stay there undetected for a very long time, at times up to several months or even years. And that is exactly what you do not want. Prompt diagnosis and immediate control of blood glucose is vital to prevent complications.

As far as possible, we should aim at preventing diabetes in the community as a whole. If you have a strong genetic background of the disease or are among those who cannot, for any reason, follow healthy lifestyle guidelines, you may not be able to prevent diabetes. In such a situation, you must aim to detect diabetes soon after its onset and begin treating it immediately. Ideally, go in for the relevant tests as soon as you cross the age of thirty years. If you understand the information on the legacy effect or metabolic memory, which we discussed in Chapter 2, you will appreciate the need for early diagnosis and prompt treatment.

However, even if you are perfectly healthy and do not have a family history of diabetes, it is advisable to go in for laboratory tests in the following situations:

1. If you exhibit symptoms such as excessive thirst or urination, or both, weight loss, tiredness, itchy skin or lesions in private parts (women) or foreskin (men).

2. If you have eczema-like skin disorders (common on the upper surface of one's feet and around the ankles) and recurrent boils, or if your wounds heal very slowly.
3. If you suffer from high blood pressure, coronary artery disease, peripheral neuropathy (which makes your palms and soles tingle or go numb) and peripheral vascular disease (which causes cramps in legs and calves when you walk).
4. If you suffer from tuberculosis.
5. If you develop cataract prematurely, before the age of fifty years.
6. If you are about to go in for any kind of surgery.
7. If you have a bad obstetric history of abortion, stillbirth or overweight newborns (needless to say, this applies to women).

Last but not the least, let me reiterate that every person, whether perfectly healthy or not, must get tested for diabetes after turning thirty. The whole idea is to catch diabetes the earliest you can, much before any complications set in, so that you can promptly control blood glucose and prevent many of the complications. In the process, some of you may be diagnosed with pre-diabetes; if so, you will have the opportunity to make the transition to a healthier, wiser, more prudent lifestyle and thus postpone or, better still, prevent the onset of diabetes.

WHAT IS PRE-DIABETES?

In some people, fasting blood glucose values and/or post-prandial blood glucose values are a bit higher than those in normal people but lower than the minimal values that would classify them as diabetics. These people are pre-diabetics because they are on the way to becoming diabetics. Every year, about 5 per cent of pre-diabetics cross over into the diabetic range.

Classification by Blood Glucose Values (in mg%)

	Normal	Pre-diabetes	Diabetes
Fasting	Up to 100	100–125	126 and above
2 hours after 75 gm glucose load	Up to 140	140–199	200 and above

4

HOW CAN I GET TESTED FOR DIABETES?

To zero in on the most effective therapy for your diabetic condition, it is important to first definitively diagnose your condition. The diagnosis of diabetes is usually very straightforward, particularly in type 1 diabetes, where the symptoms are obvious and dramatic, such as excessive thirst, excessive urination, weight loss and extreme exhaustion. In such cases, merely one confirmatory blood glucose estimation is enough to confirm the diagnosis. If random blood glucose (tested any time in the day, irrespective of food intake) is 200 mg% or over, it is definitely diabetes.

Type 2 diabetes is more insidious but if the symptoms are evident and specific diabetic complications (such as retinopathy or sensory neuropathy) are also seen, then it too requires only a confirmatory test. However, more often than not, the symptoms in type 2 diabetes are less obvious and that is why sensitive and specific tests are needed. Urine glucose testing is not adequate, so positive results should always be followed up with blood glucose estimation. In the past, when laboratory facilities to examine blood glucose were either not widely available or not affordable, presence of sugar in urine was used as a diagnostic criterion to establish the presence of diabetes.

DIAGNOSING DIABETES

1. Blood glucose estimation
2. Glycosylated haemoglobin or Haemoglobin A1C (HbA1c) estimation
3. Oral Glucose Tolerance (OGT) test
4. Test for gestational diabetes

Test 1: Blood Glucose Estimation

The preferred method to diagnose diabetes mellitus is to measure the concentration of glucose in the blood. Enzymatic methods (glucose oxidase, glucose dehydrogenase or hexokinase), which specifically measure blood glucose, should be preferred over older, non-enzymatic methods, which measure all the sugars in the blood. The resulting values may differ, depending on whether the blood is taken from a capillary (say, via a finger prick) or a vein, and whether the whole blood is tested or only the plasma. All these factors should be considered while interpreting the results. Most laboratories give information about the method of estimation and the type of blood tested. Unless specified otherwise, all the values mentioned in this book are for venous plasma glucose, the global standard for blood glucose estimation.

Values for Normal Persons

Time of test	Glucose (mg%)
Fasting	<100
2 hours after 75 gm glucose load	<140

The diagnosis of diabetes is established if any one of the following conditions is met:

- Random blood glucose level over 200 mg% in the presence of classic symptoms of diabetes such as excessive thirst, excessive urination, weight loss and severe exhaustion
- Elevated fasting glucose on more than one occasion (see table below)

Type of blood tested	Glucose (mg%)
Venous plasma	>126
Venous whole blood	>110
Capillary whole blood	>110

- Elevated plasma glucose concentration, two hours after ingestion of 75 gm of glucose orally, on more than one occasion (see table below)

Type of blood tested	Glucose (mg%)
Venous plasma	>200
Venous whole blood	>180
Capillary whole blood	>200

If one uses fasting blood glucose as the sole criterion to diagnose diabetes, it is likely to be under-diagnosed because post-glucose ingestion values are more sensitive than fasting values. However, since more people are willing to undergo a simpler and less time-consuming test such as fasting blood glucose estimation, it will serve the purpose of identifying the maximum number of diabetics in the community. (About 50 per cent of the diabetics in the US are not aware of their condition, because they do not show any of the classic symptoms and they have never taken a routine blood glucose test.)

Using a glucometer to estimate capillary blood glucose level is an excellent tool for day-to-day control but if you get a high glucose value, do not get alarmed. Instead, confirm the levels by going in for a laboratory test.

Test 2: Glycosylated Haemoglobin or Haemoglobin A1C (HbA1c) Estimation

HbA1c is a new diagnostic blood test for diabetes. HbA1c is a component of haemoglobin and is measured as a percentage of total haemoglobin. (An HbA1c level of 7 per cent means that 7 per cent of the haemoglobin comprises HbA1c component.) This test estimates average blood glucose level over the previous ninety days. While blood glucose level indicates the control status at the precise moment of drawing the blood sample, HbA1c level indicates average blood glucose control over the said period. HbA1c is considered the gold standard to assess long-term control over blood glucose in diabetics. Non-diabetics have HbA1c in the range of 4–6 per cent; values in the 6–7 per cent range in known diabetics are considered to reflect desirable control over the earlier twelve weeks.

A blood glucose test conveys the control at the particular point in time when blood is collected. It can fluctuate with time, depending on changes in how much you eat, when you eat, if and how much you exercise, what medications you are on, etc. Even a diabetic who is usually well controlled can show high blood glucose level if he misses his anti-diabetic medication on the day or eve of the test. If the treating doctor does not know this when he does a follow-up examination, he just might increase the patient's anti-diabetic medication, a totally unnecessary step.

It is wise to get your HbA1c test every three months to assess long-term control over the preceding twelve weeks. Since it represents the average blood glucose levels over the past twelve weeks, it does not significantly change even after you make the occasional slip in medication or perhaps have one of those Sunday eating binges. It is thus a more reliable indicator of long-term blood glucose control and a more reliable predictor of complications of diabetes than blood glucose estimation.

Since January 2010, the American Diabetes Association (ADA) has started to recommend HbA1c estimation as an additional option for initial diagnosis of diabetes. Values above 6.5 per cent are considered as diagnostic of diabetes. Among the reasons for this recommendation are the facts that blood can be collected any time of the day, irrespective of fasting or fed status, and there is also no need for immediate processing after the blood is collected.

Test 3: Oral Glucose Tolerance (OGT) Test

OGT is an elaborate test. First, your blood will be collected in a fasting state. Then, you will be asked to ingest 75 gm of glucose dissolved in water, and after that your blood glucose level will be measured at half-hour intervals for two hours.

Here are the guidelines for this test, addressed to pathologists:

1. Do not test if not necessary, such as in cases of overt diabetes or where the condition can be confirmed by less intensive testing. Perform this test for patients with borderline blood glucose values, who therefore need very precise diagnoses. This test can also be administered for research purposes.
2. Administer OGT in the morning after three days of normal, unrestricted diet and physical activity.
3. Ensure that the person being tested has been fasting for at least eight hours but not more than sixteen hours.
4. Make sure the person is seated and does not smoke during the test.
5. Variable loading doses of glucose: adults 75 gm; children 1.75 gm per kg body weight up to maximum 75 gm.

Test 4: Diagnosis of Gestational Diabetes

There are stringent criteria to diagnose gestational diabetes mellitus (GD), which appears during pregnancy, because of special clinical features and considerations. Recognizing that this condition is generally devoid of symptoms, the current recommendation is that all pregnant women must be screened for GD between the twenty-fourth and twenty-eighth weeks of pregnancy.

At least three different diagnostic criteria are used by different authorities. We will adhere to the following recommendations of the International Association of Diabetes and Pregnancy Study Groups, stated in 2010 and adopted by the ADA in 2011.

Diagnosis of Gestational Diabetes: Threshold Values

Glucose value	mg%
Fasting plasma glucose	92
1 hour after 75 gm oral glucose load	180
2 hours after 75 gm oral glucose load	153

Note: GD is diagnosed if one or more values are equal to or greater than the threshold.

Apart from this method, physicians and diabetologists in India also follow the World Health Organization's (WHO) definition: GD is diagnosed when plasma glucose equals or exceeds 140 mg% two hours after 75 gm glucose load.

Of course, if you have any of the following conditions, you must not wait for the twenty-fourth week! You must get screened for diabetes at the very beginning of your pregnancy.

1. Bad obstetric history (abortion, stillbirth, etc.)
2. Gestational diabetes in an earlier pregnancy
3. Known condition of diabetes
4. Diabetes in first-degree relatives (parents, siblings)
5. Obesity

Subtypes of Pre-Diabetes

Impaired glucose tolerance (IGT)

In many people, after the 75 gm glucose load, blood glucose values fall between clear normal range on one side and clear diabetic range on the other. Neither normal nor diabetic, these people are labelled as having IGT or pre-diabetes. It is like a transit port, from where you can move in either direction. If a person with IGT goes in for regular physical exercise and prudent planning of meals, his blood glucose can be normalized. Yet, IGT is also the final port of call before a person enters the clearly diabetic zone. Many people with IGT already exhibit common disorders associated with diabetes such as high blood pressure, obesity, high fat levels in the blood and coronary artery disease. Do not take IGT lightly at all. Every year, about 5 per cent of people with IGT develop diabetes.

To diagnose IGT, two criteria must be met:
1. Fasting glucose level must be below the value diagnostic for diabetes (<126 mg%).

2. Blood glucose level two hours after 75 gm oral glucose intake must be between normal and diabetic values (140–200 mg%).

Impaired fasting glucose (IFG)

In this condition, fasting blood glucose level is somewhere between the normal range and the diabetic range (100–126 mg%). IFG has the same implications as those of IGT and is considered a pre-diabetic stage. Some people have isolated IFG or IGT while others have both at the same time.

How Should I Prepare for a Blood Glucose Test?

You undergo blood glucose tests initially to help diagnose diabetes and then to assess control of blood glucose levels. Your doctor studies these reports, gauges your current status and makes appropriate changes in the treatment plan. The idea is to bring you back on track in case your blood glucose control has derailed so that you can avert complications and maintain quality of life. While studying your blood glucose report, your doctor assumes that you have followed your diet, exercise and medication regimens honestly for several days before the test, and more so on the eve of the tests as well as the day of the test, right up to the post-prandial test. If you deviate from your schedules around blood glucose testing time, your report—even though technically correct— will misguide your doctor and he may make inappropriate decisions about your treatment.

Here are some common mistakes:

1. Instead of your regular dinner at 9 p.m., you indulged in a heavy dinner followed by dessert at midnight, since it is a dear friend's party that you cannot possibly avoid. And then, since you were very busy that day, you called the pathologist's technician home at 6.30 a.m. the very next day to collect your blood sample for, mind you, fasting blood glucose level! As you can imagine, the level will be much higher than your usual fasting level.

2. You wanted a good blood glucose report to put an end to your spouse's nagging about your overeating. So, you ate only half your lunch! You will get a better than usual post-prandial blood glucose report but, in reality, you will end up deceiving not only your wife but also yourself.

3. Your usual lunchtime is 1 p.m., so blood should be drawn at 3 p.m. (exactly two hours after the beginning of lunch) to estimate post-lunch blood glucose. However, the laboratory is closed between 1 and 4 p.m. so the pathologist's assistant advises you to eat a 'double breakfast' at 10 a.m. and come for the blood test at noon. He believes that the 'double breakfast' will simulate lunch taken at 1 p.m. but that is far from true. Your post-prandial blood glucose report will deviate from your usual figures.

If you have missed or deviated from the previous day's anti-diabetic medication, particularly in the evening, your fasting blood glucose will convey wrong information. If you have deviated from the morning dose on the morning of post-prandial blood glucose estimation, the test result will convey wrong information.

> A blood glucose test is not a boring chore. Be careful. If you do not take precautions and if it is not done properly, the doctor may get incorrect information about your condition and treat you inappropriately!

Remember to take all your usual medications on the eve and day of the test. Some people deliberately omit their morning medication on the day of the test, all because they want to study their 'natural' control. Well, rise and shine! There is nothing 'natural' about diabetes. When your doctor advises you to take anti-diabetic medications, he has already verified that your diabetes has reached a state where you need medication to control blood glucose. These medications stay active in your body for a few hours, after which they are eliminated. Around the time their levels start dropping to ineffective levels, you are due for the next dose. If you miss that next dose, your blood glucose will 'naturally' go up.

If, due to an oversight, you miss taking your medication on the test day and realize it in time, postpone the post-prandial blood glucose test to the next day and ensure that you maintain your schedules. It is perfectly all right to test fasting and post-prandial blood glucose at a gap of one or two days.

CHECKLIST TO PREPARE FOR BLOOD GLUCOSE ESTIMATION TESTS

- Ensure that you stick to your usual time, amount and type of food and take your regular medicines at the regular time the day before the test.
- Fast overnight for at least eight hours. You can drink water if you want.
- Get your fasting blood sample drawn before 9 a.m. If you usually exercise before breakfast, do so as usual on the day of the test.
- For random or post-prandial tests, take your breakfast and any pre- or post-breakfast medicines as usual.
- Take your mid-morning snack and lunch at the usual time and in the usual amount. Also take your pre- and post-lunch medicines as usual.
- Get a post-prandial blood test exactly two hours after you started lunch.

Some doctors prefer post-breakfast blood glucose estimation instead of post-lunch. As long as it is done properly, it is fine to substitute. Make sure that your doctor knows which one you have got done.

5

HOW MANY TYPES OF DIABETES ARE THERE?

Diabetes mellitus is a condition in which blood glucose levels are higher than they should be. It is not a single disease but a syndrome, or a group of diseases, with elevated blood glucose as a common factor. There are four types of diabetes:

1. Type 1 diabetes
2. Type 2 diabetes
3. Secondary diabetes
4. Gestational diabetes

Type 1 Diabetes Mellitus

About 2 per cent of Indian diabetics belong to this subclass, earlier known as insulin dependent diabetes mellitus (IDDM). Type 1 DM develops when the body's insulin-producing beta cells in the pancreas are destroyed by the defence system, which fails to differentiate between invading viruses and the body's own cells. Thus, it may follow a recognizable episode of viral infection in some cases. In others, there is no evident underlying cause.

Type 1 DM is usually acute at the onset—it develops very swiftly, usually in childhood or adolescence. In these patients, insulin is not produced at all, so their survival is dependent on insulin administered daily via injections. If their insulin is withdrawn for a substantial time period, they will develop diabetic ketoacidosis and possibly go into a diabetic coma, which is fatal. These patients should never discontinue insulin, even during sick days, because even when they are not eating or drinking, their liver still produces large quantities of glucose while there is no 'natural' insulin around to suppress it.

Remember that type 1 DM is a relatively rare subtype of diabetes in India. Not all young and insulin-requiring diabetics are necessarily insulin-dependent. Some of them could be pancreatic diabetics or have maturity onset diabetes of young (MODY), which presents itself at a young age.

Type 2 Diabetes Mellitus

Subtype: Adults

The most common subtype of diabetes, this has been known earlier as non-insulin dependent diabetes mellitus (NIDDM) and maturity onset diabetes (MOD) because it typically sets in during middle age. As many as 96 per cent of Indian diabetics have this condition.

Type 2 diabetes is partly hereditary and partly environmental. The nature of inheritance is complex and multiple genes are involved. Those who inherit the genes for diabetes have a limited capacity to produce insulin. If they develop insulin resistance due to environmental factors (lack of exercise, overeating, unhealthy diet causing obesity, etc.), at some point, their pancreas fails to cope with the increased insulin demand, thus leading to relative insulin deficiency and hence diabetes. However, it is not necessary to be obese to develop diabetes. In fact, more often than not, diabetics in India are non-obese.

In some people, the hereditary factor is much more dominant than environmental factors; insufficient insulin formation leading to actual (not relative) insulin deficiency is the dominant cause. In brief, diabetes and obesity often coexist, but not all obese persons are diabetics and vice versa. However, it is interesting that in the case of twins, who have a common inheritance, the obese twin is more likely to develop diabetes. If heredity is the dominant contributor, the normal-weight twin will develop diabetes much later than his overweight counterpart and require lesser medication than the latter. If environmental factors are predominant, the normal-weight twin may not develop diabetes till the end of his life, while the overweight counterpart may develop it in middle age.

Symptoms

Type 2 DM usually develops in middle age and symptoms are gradual. Initially, patients do not show any symptoms, and this phase can last for as long as five years. During this phase, diabetes may be accidentally detected in some people via a pre-employment check-up or pre-surgical check-up or pre-insurance check-up. In some, it is detected when they consult a doctor for some other medical condition such as high blood pressure or heart disease. Those who are not diagnosed gradually develop symptoms such as excessive thirst, excessive urination, weight loss despite good appetite, itching of private parts (in women), foreskin lesions (in men), tiredness, tingling and numbness in the feet and fungal skin infections (particularly in the groin and web spaces between toes).

Some mild type 2 diabetics can control their condition through diet and exercise, and do not require medication. However, most type 2 diabetics do need medicines in addition to—not instead of—diet and exercise. Severe diabetics whose beta cells have lost the capacity to produce insulin in any significant amount require insulin injections to control blood glucose but not for immediate survival. They are called 'insulin requiring' (but not dependent) type 2 diabetics.

Whether a diabetic requires a non-medication approach or medication in addition to dietary control and physical exercise or insulin depends on the residual capacity of his beta cells to produce insulin. Since diabetes is a progressive disease, the capacity of the pancreas to produce insulin declines over time. Even though we have medicines to bring down blood glucose, scientists have not yet found a drug to halt progressive decline of insulin-producing capacity, so the requirements of diabetics change with time. No two diabetics are similar in type and severity of symptoms or type and dosage of medicines (including insulin). Moreover, the symptoms and medicinal requirements of a diabetic are continually changing, depending on several factors including duration of diabetes, diet, physical activity, associated conditions and so on. A diabetic should never compare himself with other diabetics, and should also avoid comparisons between his own past and current status.

Subtype: Children and adolescents

Till the 1990s, type 2 diabetes was considered exclusive to adults, especially middle-aged adults; in fact, it was officially known as maturity onset diabetes or MOD. Over the last decade, however, more and more cases have been detected in children and adolescents. What is disturbing is that its prevalence is rising rapidly. Such cases were first detected in western countries and soon started appearing in India as well. In the US, till a decade ago, less than 3 per cent of diabetic children had type 2 diabetes; now the figure is a whopping 45 per cent. In Japan, 80 per cent of children with diabetes have type 2 diabetes. Such precise figures are not available for India yet but it is quite likely that our figures are closely following those of the advanced countries.

Clinical features

The common age of onset is during adolescence and teens, typically between the ages of twelve and eighteen years. The clinical features are similar to those of adult type 2 diabetics. Most patients are obese; even morbid obesity is not rare. There are signs of insulin resistance, such as acanthosis nigricans (dark purplish or black skin lesions, usually at the nape). They have a strong family history of type 2 diabetes. Like their adult counterparts, these children develop symptoms very gradually in the onset. Some common symptoms are weight loss, lethargy, tiredness, excessive thirst and urination and itching.

Causes

The rising prevalence of type 2 diabetes in children and adolescents is mainly due to the rising obesity in this age group. While the last century saw a gradual increase in obesity in young people, the rate of increase has accelerated tremendously over the 1990s and 2000s. A recent survey done among Chennai's urban population by A. Ramachandran on 4,700 children aged thirteen to eighteen years found that 22 per cent, 15 per cent and 4.5 per cent of the children from high, middle and low economic classes, respectively, were overweight.[1] With the socio-economic flux and rampant globalization, children's food habits are also changing rapidly, whether it is dining in restaurants frequently or eating fibre-sparse and energy-dense foods, such as bread made of maida instead of roti made of atta at home. And what with aggressive marketing schemes and attractive giveaways, children insist on jumbo-sized food items and tantalizingly priced multi-unit packs that make us buy more and make them eat more. To compound this dietary indiscipline is the physical inactivity prompted by the television and the Internet. No wonder children are getting obese!

---

1 A. Ramchandran, 'Obesity in school children in Chennai', *Diabetes Research and Clinical Practice* 57: 185–90.

A TYPICAL CASE OF TYPE 2 DIABETES IN CHILDHOOD

Rajesh is fifteen. He is 150 cm tall and weighs 72 kg. Thus, his body mass index is 32, which falls in the moderately obese category as per WHO benchmarks. Rajesh is very fond of playing computer games and spends about ninety minutes every day surfing the Internet. While he is at it, he relishes his burgers and French fries. Of course, he has no time for outdoor sports or any physical activity. Six months ago, the child was diagnosed with diabetes when he showed symptoms of excessive urination, weight loss and itching. Both his parents had developed diabetes in their forties.

At the time of his diagnosis, Rajesh did not have ketones in his urine and did not appear dehydrated or acutely ill. Moreover, he was obese and had a strong family history of type 2 diabetes. Thus, his doctor suspected that Rajesh's diabetes was not type 1 diabetes, which typically sets in during childhood, but type 2 diabetes, which usually appears in adults. Rajesh was referred to a diabetologist who did blood tests to confirm that Rajesh is indeed a type 2 diabetic, even though he is only fifteen.

Major Types of Diabetes Mellitus

	Type 1	Type 2
Age at diagnosis	Childhood, adolescence (8–15 years)	Middle age (in the West, 4th and 5th decades of life; in India, 3rd and 4th decades of life)
Onset	Rapid	Slow
Symptoms	Classic: excessive thirst, excessive urination, weight loss, extreme exhaustion	Often absent or non-specific
Insulin deficiency	Absolute; patient cannot survive without insulin	Relative; in most patients, it can be controlled via diet and oral medication in initial years; many require insulin later in life
Prevalence (among all diabetics in India)	2%	96%

Stress diabetes: A temporary class of Type 2 diabetes

Some people, particularly those who have inherited genes for diabetes, develop diabetes temporarily during periods of severe stress, such as a major accident, administration of corticosteroids, a major infection like extensive tuberculosis or a major brain disease like a tumour or stroke. Once the stressful condition subsides, their blood glucose values return to normal levels so they do not require medication to control blood glucose. However, such people should always remember that they are more prone to develop diabetes in later years even in the absence of stress. They should get their blood glucose estimated at yearly intervals even if they are feeling perfectly healthy, and focus on preventing the onset of permanent diabetes.

Most other people do not develop temporary stress diabetes even during stressful periods because they have robust pancreatic capacity to rise to the demand of extra insulin during stress.

Secondary Diabetes

There are some rare conditions associated with or leading to diabetes, as listed below. Together, these are responsible for about 2 per cent of diabetics in India.

- Genetic defects of beta cell function
- Genetic defects in insulin action
- Diseases of exocrine pancreas (pancreatitis, fibro calculus pancreatic diseases)
- Endocrine disorders (Cushing's syndrome, acromegaly, thyrotoxicosis)
- Drug- or chemical-induced diabetes (thiazide)
- Infections (congenital rubella)
- Immune-mediated diabetes
- Other genetic syndromes (Down's syndrome)

Gestational Diabetes

Diabetes first diagnosed during pregnancy is called gestational diabetes (GD). It occurs in about 4 per cent of pregnancies in western countries. It is seen more commonly in India. In a study done on 4151 pregnant women from low- and middle-class strata in Tamil Nadu, 17.8 per cent women from urban areas, 13.8 per cent women from semi-urban areas and 9.9 per cent women from rural areas were found to have GD. This condition results from the insulin resistance of pregnancy interacting with beta cell defects. Usually blood glucose is normalized after delivery. Since significant insulin resistance of pregnancy develops only in the third trimester, GD sets in only in this period. The presence of high blood glucose in early pregnancy usually indicates pre-existing type 1 or type 2 DM. Women with GD are at higher risk of developing type 2 DM at a later stage in life.

Pre-diabetes States

Impaired glucose tolerance or IGT

In this condition, post-prandial blood glucose levels are in the zone between normal values on one side and clearly diabetic values on the other. Many of these people develop diabetes after some time. However, with prudent lifestyle management including diet control and exercise, many of them revert to non-diabetic status.

Impaired fasting glucose or IFG

In this condition, fasting blood glucose is between the normal and diabetic range, which is 100–126 mg%. Like impaired glucose tolerance, it is a pre-diabetic condition.

Some people have isolated IGT or IFG, while some have a combination of both.

Older Classification of Diabetes

The above-mentioned classification of diabetes was initially put up by the ADA in 1997 and subsequently adapted by the WHO in 1998. The earlier classification, in use till 1997, had a subtype called malnutrition-related diabetes or pancreatic diabetes. Patients earlier classified in this type are seen in many developing countries like India, particularly in the southern and eastern states. Usually, teenagers and young adults are affected in their second or third decades. These children are usually malnourished and they require relatively large doses of insulin for control. At the same time, if they discontinue insulin, they will not go into diabetic ketoacidosis unless severe stressful conditions coexist. Hence these patients are insulin-requiring but not insulin-dependent. Pancreatic diabetes has two subtypes.

Fibro calculus pancreatic diabetes (FCPD)

This develops after chronic pancreatitis associated with destruction of beta cells and stone formation in the pancreatic duct. The symptoms are recurrent and severe upper abdominal pain. Abdominal X-ray and ultrasonography reveal pancreatic stones and clinches the diagnosis. FCPD is now reclassified under 'other specific types' because it is secondary to pancreatic destruction.

Protein deficient diabetes mellitus (PDDM)

Many of these patients have suffered from severe protein deficiency in their infancy and early childhood leading to damaged beta cells in the pancreas. Many PDDM patients have current or old signs of undernutrition. According to the current classification, PDDM does not warrant a separate class and is included in type 2 diabetes.

DIABETICS IN INDIA

- India has the world's second largest number of diabetics, after China.
- The percentage of type 2 diabetics among the diabetic population in India is higher than in the developed countries, except developed Asian countries like Japan.
- In India, type 2 diabetes presents itself at least ten to fifteen years earlier than in western countries.
- Obesity is not as commonly associated with type 2 diabetics in India compared with the West. Despite this, insulin resistance is quite common. Indians tend

to accumulate excessive fat in the abdomen, even if they are not obese. Such fat distribution—called central obesity—is more strongly associated with diabetes and heart disease than general obesity. Thus many Indians are 'thin but fat'. They are non-obese by general obesity criteria but have excessive fat deposits in the abdomen.

- The hereditary component in the development of type 2 DM is strong, particularly in south India.
- A small percentage of patients exhibit secondary diabetes following destruction of pancreas due to fibro calculus pancreatic disease. This is restricted to developing countries such as India.

6

HOW CAN I MANAGE MY DIABETES?

The surest way of managing your diabetic condition and living happily despite the disease is to know it, understand it, counter it and live an extremely disciplined life. The management of diabetes revolves around four cornerstones (see figure).

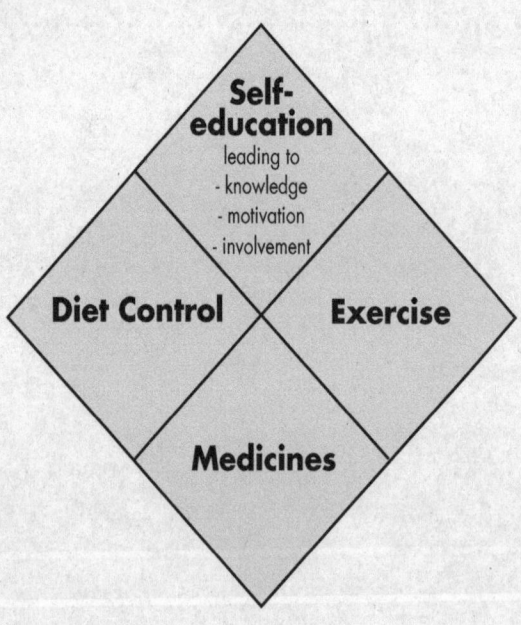

All the four modalities of management—self-education, diet control, exercise and medication—are equally important and should be implemented simultaneously. Just as a war can be won only if all three wings of a nation's armed forces (army, air force, navy) are coordinated well by their commanders, and just as a cricket match can be won only if all four departments (batting, bowling, fielding, captaincy) are perfectly in sync, the war against diabetes can be won easily only if the patient is motivated, involved and informed enough to simultaneously deploy his three weapons—physical exercise, diet and medication—in coordination. He must understand that there is no alternative to establishing his diabetic status as early as possible and maintaining strict glycaemic control.

LIVING EASY WITH DIABETES FOR OVER FORTY YEARS: THE ULTIMATE CASE STUDY

The real-life success story of a woman who has lived her life totally free of any complications of diabetes for over four decades

Dr Shaila P. Bhatwadekar is sixty-nine years old and has had diabetes for forty-four years. She retired nine years ago as the chief of biochemistry at the Central Institute for Cotton Research.

Both her parents as well as two maternal uncles were diabetics. Her parents lived disciplined lives. They were regular with their diet, exercise and medication, and always kept their weight in control. They lived long and high quality lives, without any handicaps associated with diabetic complications. So, while Shaila inherited the gene for diabetes from both parents, she also 'inherited' a strong sense of discipline from them.

Shaila became a diabetic very early, at the age of twenty-five years. For a whopping forty-four years, she has succeeded in keeping at bay all the complications of diabetes, and is still going strong. It is not an easy accomplishment, and Shaila has achieved this goal through sheer hard work.

She walks for 5 km every morning, strictly adheres to her diet plan and is very strict with her medication regimen. She goes for regular follow-up visits to her diabetologist every three months and is never lax about the periodic laboratory investigation schedule drawn up by her doctor. She has not only preserved all her laboratory investigation reports meticulously but has also tabulated them by year and by investigation type. She has been persistently achieving her blood glucose, blood pressure and cholesterol goals.

Always eager to learn more about diabetes, Shaila never misses an opportunity to attend educational seminars on the subject. She has been my patient for the last two decades. I often call her to give pep talks to encourage my other patients at yearly get-togethers. In fact, over the last few years, she has given several 'How Did I Achieve It?' talks at interactive educational seminars to guide and encourage other patients.

Shaila's is an extremely rare case because despite having diabetes for over four decades, she does not have any complications that inevitably accompany it. What is the secret of her success? She says she has no secrets, only a success formula, and here it is:

- Persistently acquire and update your knowledge on diabetes
- Use this knowledge intelligently to achieve your set goals
- Maintain a strictly disciplined lifestyle
- Comply with your medication regimen religiously and unfailingly
- Regularly follow up with the doctors to verify blood glucose control and status of various organs

By following this formula, Shaila has achieved a high-quality and totally independent life despite her potentially debilitating condition.

Shaila has been living easy with diabetes for a long time. If Shaila can do it, why can't you?

In the next four chapters, let us understand more about each of these modalities, namely, planning your meals, planning your physical exercise regimen and planning your intake of oral medication as well as insulin.

7

MANAGING DIABETES: PLANNING MEALS

Planning one's meals and a judicious selection of food type and quantity is a vital and primary step in managing diabetes. In fact, food regimentation and regular exercise in combination are sufficient to control blood glucose in mild diabetics. Those dependent on insulin or medicines to lower blood glucose should never neglect meal planning because their diabetologist decides the dosage of their insulin/medication very carefully on the basis of their food intake, and misalignment of the two can cause complications such as hypoglycaemia or hyperglycaemia.

I try to avoid the term 'diet' because people interpret it variously, more often than not as a restriction in food quantity across the board. It has negative, restrictive or unfriendly connotations. In fact, diabetics who have an ideal body weight need not restrict the number of calories they consume in a day. What they need to do is to take frequent but smaller meals; avoid refined sugars and fatty food; and go for ample rough cereals and vegetables to get adequate fibre into their systems. If you understand the basic principles of sensible eating, you can consume the same food as the rest of your family. A diabetic does not require any specially prepared meal. Also, like normal people, you can, and should, keep changing your meal plan to break the monotony.

Not only diabetics but all of us must consume well-balanced food to promote growth in our formative years, maintain our bodily functions and compensate for the wear and tear of our tissues. While charting your daily meal plan, your objectives should be to (1) provide the required number of calories to create energy and attain/maintain ideal body weight and (2) plan a well-balanced meal featuring proteins, carbohydrates, fats, fibres, vitamins and minerals in optimum proportions.

Overweight people should cut down on the total number of calories and consume less than their daily requirement so that the extra fat stored under the skin and in the abdominal cavity is burnt to bridge the gap between calories consumed and calories required. This way, they can shed their extra weight. In many diabetics, particularly the obese, insulin deficiency is only relative, not absolute. Some actually produce more insulin than normal people. However, because of their obesity, tissue response to insulin is much lower than in normal persons—they have insulin resistance. When the extra weight is shed, tissue response to insulin improves, so blood glucose is lowered. In other words, when obesity is corrected, your tissues get extra mileage out of the body's own insulin.

A balanced meal plan contains all the constituents of food in optimum proportions.

Carbohydrates

Carbohydrates form the main source of energy. Cereals and cereal-based foods supply complex carbohydrates while sugar, honey, jam, etc. provide simple carbohydrates. About 60–65 per cent of your body's energy requirement should be met by carbohydrates, mainly complex ones. You should avoid simple sugar and any items containing it. Foods made with complex carbohydrates (rice, bread, chapati) form the bulk of our meals. These are converted into glucose gradually so their consumption does not result in any sudden rise in blood glucose levels. However, you should shun simple sugar (sucrose) as it gets converted into glucose very rapidly.

Proteins

Proteins are essential for growth as well as repair of tissues. Milk and milk products, egg white, meat, fish, nuts and pulses are rich sources of proteins. About 15–20 per cent of calories you need every day should come from proteins. Adult diabetics should consume about 0.8 gm of proteins per 1 kg of body weight. However, diabetics with associated kidney damage should consume smaller amounts of protein, as per their doctor's advice.

Fats

Fats are important for energy storage. They are vital constituents of cell membranes, and consist of fatty acids and glycerides. Depending on the type of fatty acid they contain, fats can be one of three types:

1. *Saturated Fats*: Animal fat and fat from milk, milk products and vanaspati[1] are all rich in saturated fat. Animal fats are also rich in cholesterol. Consuming too much saturated fats and cholesterol will harm your health by hardening and narrowing your blood vessels. Saturated fats should provide only one-third of the energy you derive from all fats, which in turn should be about 20 per cent of total energy intake. Cooking oils rich in saturated fats are coconut oil, palm kernel oil, vanaspati and ghee.

2. *Monounsaturated Fats*: Oils from groundnuts, mustard, palm (red palm oil, palmolein), rice bran, sesame and olives provide monounsaturated fats. You should aim at deriving one-third of total fat-derived energy from monounsaturated fats.

3. *Polyunsaturated Fats*: Mustard oil, safflower oil, sunflower oil, corn oil, soybean oil and cottonseed oil are some rich sources of polyunsaturated fats. These should provide the remaining one-third of energy from fats.

Essential fatty acids

Some fatty acids, such as Omega 6 (w6) and Omega 3 (w3), cannot be made in the body, which is why you need to

---

1 Vanaspati is hydrogenated vegetable oil. When vegetable oil is hydrogenated, it is converted from liquid to solid form, thus appearing like ghee, and its fatty acids are converted from polyunsaturated to saturated form. Food cooked in vanaspati keeps for longer, as it resists oxidation. Also, vanaspati is cheaper than ghee so it is used commonly.

assimilate them from food. The fats we consume provide these fatty acids but each type of fat has w6 and w3 in different proportions. The ideal proportion is w6:w3 = 4:1.

Certain oils rich in polyunsaturated fatty acids, such as safflower and sunflower oil, are aggressively marketed as safe or healthy oils, in that their consumption does not lead to a rise in blood cholesterol. Media advertisements indirectly claim that you can consume large quantities of these oils. Remember, however, that all oils provide the same number of calories per unit volume. So the more you eat, the more calories you take in. Moreover, these 'safe' oils have a rather unfavourable w6:w3 ratio of about 150:1. Contrary to what advertisements may have you believe, consuming these oils in excessive amounts is not safe at all.

For the ideal w6:w3 ratio, use cooking mediums such as mustard oil, coconut oil or ghee. Ghee and coconut oil are richer in saturated fats, so use them in smaller quantities. Fish oil is a very good source of w3 fatty acids. If you don't eat fish, you can go with one to three capsules of fish oil, though it has not yet been proved that capsulated fish oil is as good as natural fish in terms of preventing cardiovascular complications.

FATTY FUNDAMENTALS

- Limit your fat intake to 20 per cent of the total energy you need.

- Consume saturated, monounsaturated and poly-unsaturated fats in equal amounts.
- Don't have any fat or oil in unlimited quantities—no fat or oil is 'totally safe'.
- Don't shun ghee totally. In fact, since it provides the ideal w6:w3 ratio of essential fatty acids compared with oils rich in polyunsaturated fatty acids, like sunflower oil, it is good for you to have a little bit of ghee, say ½ to 1 tsp daily.
- Mustard oil and coconut oil have good w3:w6 ratio and are recommended for cooking. You can mix them with sunflower oil. Other sources of w3 fatty acids are fish liver oil, flax seeds, walnuts, wheat, bajra, black gram, cowpea, kidney bean, green leafy vegetables and fenugreek.
- Limit consumption of cooking oil to ½ kg per month—this works out to 4 tsp daily.

Fibre

From the indigestible plant cell components of our food comes the very important diet element called fibre. Fibres can be of two types.

Water-insoluble fibre

Water-insoluble fibre, which adds bulk to your food and has a laxative effect, thus helping you avoid constipation.

Wholewheat, whole grains, wheat bran, corn bran, brown rice, whole pulses, nuts and seeds, grapes and fruit and root vegetable skin are rich in this fibre.

Water-soluble fibre

Water-soluble fibre absorbs water to swell up and makes you feel full, thus helping you control your food intake and reduce weight. Oatmeal, lentils, apples, oranges, pears, beans and flax seeds are rich in this fibre.

A traditional Indian vegetarian diet—rich in vegetables, fruit and cereals—provides adequate fibre; hence supplementary medicated fibre preparations (usually rather expensive) are not required. You can provide adequate fibre-rich, natural food items for the entire (average-sized) family at a reasonable cost.

WHY MUST I INCLUDE FIBRE IN MY DIET?

- Fibre slows down the digestion of carbohydrates into glucose, and its absorption, so there is no sharp post-meal rise in blood glucose.
- High fibre intake helps reduce the levels of blood cholesterol and triglycerides, both likely to be high in diabetics, and both potential risk factors for heart disease.

- Especially with water-soluble fibre, you feel full and avoid eating more food. This helps you control your weight and, thus, your blood glucose.
- Consuming water-insoluble fibre prevents constipation. By preventing chronic constipation, chances of large bowel cancer are reduced.

Water

Apart from being absolutely essential for survival, it is an important constituent of all foods. You need a sufficient amount of water to digest your food properly and completely. People with impaired heart and kidney functions should limit their water intake because drinking too much water increases the volume of blood and, therefore, the workload on the heart. Those with failing kidneys cannot compensate by eliminating the extra water through urine.

Vitamins and Minerals

Diabetics need vitamins and minerals in the same quantities as normal people. Well-balanced meals provide you all the vitamins and minerals you need in adequate quantities. If you are on a very-low-calorie diet, take one multivitamin or B-complex capsule daily. Many diabetics are habituated to eating tablets containing vitamins B1, B6 and B12, some of them for all their lives. These are totally useless for most of them because extra quantities of these vitamins are promptly excreted through urine.

Of late, it has also become fashionable to consume large doses of vitamin D because Indians, particularly diabetics, are prone to vitamin D deficiency. The pharmaceutical industry claims that vitamin D prevents not only the complications of diabetes but indeed diabetes itself. While it is true that vitamin D deficiency is common in Indians, especially those with cardiovascular disease and diabetes, it has not yet been proved that vitamin D prevents diabetes or its complications. Thus one should not go overboard but consume it judiciously. In fact, some years ago, the Central Drugs Standard Control Organization of India placed a ceiling on the amount of each vitamin that can be added to a multivitamin formulation.

THE GOODNESS OF FRUITS

Fruits are a superb source of vitamins as well as antioxidants. You can safely eat one medium-sized fruit (roughly 200 gm) or 12–15 grapes every day. Change your fruit depending on the season and your preference. You can even have mangoes in limited quantities. Isn't that sweet news? Do take care, however, not to have too much of chikoo or very ripe banana as these contain rather high quantities of sugar.

Meal Planning

To plan your daily meal in a logical manner, ask yourself these questions:
1. What is my ideal body weight?
2. How many calories should I consume daily?
3. What is the best meal plan to deliver the calories I need?

Step 1: Calculate your ideal body weight

Measure your height in centimetres and subtract 100 (for men) or 105 (for women) from it to get a rough idea of your ideal body weight. For example, if your height is 170 cm, your ideal body weight should be around 70 kg (for men) or 61 kg (for women). Please remember that the height–weight charts that you see in many doctors' clinics are based on outdated data. Add 10 per cent to their figures to get a rough idea of ideal body weight.

While this formula yields a rough estimate, we now rely more on the body mass index (BMI), calculated by the following formula:

BMI = weight (in kg)/square of height (in m)

The normal range is 18–23 for men and 19–25 for women. If Ram is 170 cm tall and weighs 60 kg, his BMI works out as 60/1.7*1.7 = 20.8, which lies within the normal range. However, if Shyama is 155 cm tall and weighs 80 kg, her BMI works out as 80/1.55*1.55 = 33.3, which is way beyond the normal range and places her in the obese category. You should maintain your BMI in the normal range. If it rises, shed some weight.

Weight Category on the Basis of Body Mass Index

Category	BMI
Underweight	<18
Normal	18–23
Overweight	23–28
Mildly obese	28–33
Moderately obese	33–38
Morbidly obese	>38

WAIST TO HEALTH

Waist circumference is an easily measured and very useful indicator of central or upper body obesity. Central obesity is diagnosed if waist circumference at the highest point of the iliac crest (a bony prominence on the sides) is above 90 cm in men and above 80 cm in women. Even a person with normal BMI can be centrally obese. Since central obesity is more strongly associated with cardiovascular disease than general obesity, it is vital to maintain an ideal waist circumference.

Step 2: Calculate the calories you need daily

Use this table to calculate how many calories you require.

**Energy Requirement (Calories Per Day)
by Nature of Work and Weight**

Group	Sedentary	Moderate	Heavy
Overweight	20	30	35
Normal weight	30	35	40
Underweight	35	40	45–50
Bedridden patients	—	25	—

Classification of a few activities

Sedentary: Business executive, banker, writer/editor, nurse, doctor, businessman, desk worker

Moderate: Fisherman, potter, agricultural labourer, carpenter, electrician, welder, turner, industrial labourer

Heavy: Stonecutter, mine worker, woodcutter

Overweight persons should consciously consume fewer calories than their daily requirement so that the fat stored in their bodies is spent to bridge the demand–supply gap. Deepak weighs 70 kg and his BMI is 27; thus he is placed in the overweight category. He is a banker, so his work is sedentary. He should consume 70 × 20 = 1400 calories in a day. This will help him shed weight. On the other hand, growing children, pregnant and lactating women, and underweight or debilitated persons with diabetes should consume extra calories.

Step 3: Convert the calorie requirement into an ideal meal plan

To do this, you must know the composition of the various foods you eat and the calories provided by each gram of protein, carbohydrate and fat.

Cereals like rice and wheat are rich in carbohydrates, which form about 70 per cent of their weight, but poor in proteins, while pulses and lentils (dals) are comparatively richer in proteins. Commonly used vegetables are rich in carbohydrates and vitamins, as well as in micronutrients, but have negligible quantities of proteins. All these foods provide very small quantities of fat, known as 'invisible fat'. Meat and fish are rich in proteins while the former, particularly red meat, is also rich in fat. Both these are low on carbohydrates. Milk provides all the three with its fat composition varying, depending on the animal source and also whether it is processed to render it 'low fat'.

Each gram of protein and carbohydrates provides 4 calories, while each gram of fat provides 9 calories.

From Step 2, you already know the calories you require every day, so select an ideal meal plan by referring to this 'meal-planning chart'. The food exchanges are explained right after.

Please note that calorific values set out by the Planning Commission of India to measure the poverty line are 2100 calories a day for urban areas and 2400 calories a day for rural areas. However, diabetics are often overweight and are prescribed lower calories than their needs so that accumulated fat is mobilized and burnt to produce energy. This helps them reach their weight and waist circumference goals. Hence, I have given a range of plans from 1200 calories to 2400 calories.

Meal-planning Chart

Meal Units	Calories required					
	1200	1600	1800	2000	2200	2400
Morning tea/coffee (with 1/3 cup milk)	1 cup	1 cup	1 cup	1 cup	1 cup	1 cup
Breakfast						
Cereal exchange	2	2	3	3	3	4
Milk exchange	1	1	1	1	1	1
Fat exchange	½	1	1	1	1	1
Mid-morning snack						
Fruit exchange	1	1	1	1	1	1
Milk exchange	nil	nil	nil	nil	1	1
Lunch						
Cereal exchange	2	2½	3	4	4	5
Pulse exchange	1	1	1½	1½	1½	1½
Curd	50 ml	100 ml	100 ml	100 ml	100 ml	100 ml
A Group vegetables	unlimited					
B Group vegetables	1	1	1	1	1	1
Fat exchange	½	1	1	1	1	1
Afternoon snack						
Tea/coffee	1 cup	1 cup	1 cup	1 cup	1 cup	1 cup
Cereal exchange	1	2	2	2	2	2
Fat exchange	½	1	1	1	1	1

Contd...

73

... contd.

	Calories required					
Meal Units	1200	1600	1800	2000	2200	2400
Evening snack						
Fruit exchange	1	1	1	1	1	1
Milk exchange	nil	nil	nil	nil	1	1
Dinner (same as lunch)						
Bedtime						
Milk exchange	1	1	1	1	1	1

Note: 1 egg can be replaced with 1 milk exchange; ½ cereal exchange can be replaced with 1 fruit exchange in the evening and at bedtime

The food exchanges

You can and should make frequent changes to your meal plan to avoid any monotony, which can indirectly tempt you into binging now and then. Of course, while you make these changes, ensure that you maintain the total calories consumed in a day as well as the proportion of calories you derive from carbohydrates, proteins and fats. To make these changes, you should know alternatives for each item of your daily meal. For example, if you don't want a cup of cow's milk at breakfast, what else can you have? Here is a list of food exchanges to fall back on.

Cereal exchange

Each exchange provides carbohydrates 15 gm; proteins 2 gm; calories 70

One exchange = any one of the following.

Cooked rice	75 gm (3 tbsp)
Chapati	1, made with 20 gm wholewheat flour
Roti	1, made with 20 gm flour of jowar, bajra, corn, ragi
Idli	1 medium
Bread	30 gm (1½ slices)
Cornflakes	20 gm (3 tbsp)
Dosa	1 medium
Porridge	¾ cup
Marie biscuit	3

Pulses exchange

Each exchange provides carbohydrates 15 gm; proteins 6 gm; fat 1 gm; calories 91

One exchange = any one of the following

Kidney beans (rajma)	25 gm (raw weight)
Chickpeas (chholey)	25 gm (raw weight)
Black gram (kala chana)	25 gm (raw weight)
Black-eyed peas (lobhia)	25 gm (raw weight)
Green gram (mung)	25 gm (raw weight)
Red gram (masoor)	25 gm (raw weight)

Meat exchange

Each exchange provides carbohydrates nil; proteins 7 gm; fat 5 gm; calories 70

One exchange = any one of the following

Mutton	30 gm
Chicken	50 gm
Fish	60 gm
Pork	30 gm
Ham	20 gm
Beef	50 gm
Egg	50 gm (1 unit)

Milk exchange

Each exchange provides carbohydrates 7.5 gm; proteins 4.5 gm; fat 5 gm; calories 108

One exchange = any one of the following

Cow's milk	150 ml
Buffalo milk	90 ml
Skimmed milk	350 ml
Skimmed milk powder	30 gm (3 tbsp)
Buttermilk	750 ml
Curd (cow's milk)	150 ml
Cheese	30 gm

Note: Skimmed milk products are richer in proteins. The powder provides 11 gm proteins per 30 gm while the milk provides 8 gm per 350 ml.

Fruit exchange

Each exchange provides carbohydrates 10 gm; calories 40

One exchange = any one of the following

Orange	100 gm (1 medium)
Pear	90 gm (1 medium)
Apple	90 gm (1 medium)

Banana	40 gm (1 medium)
Mango	60 gm (½ small)
Watermelon	300 gm (3 slices)
Papaya	120 gm (2 slices)
Grapes	75 gm (12 units)
Guava	100 gm (1 medium)
Dried dates	5 gm (4–5 units)
Figs	100 gm (3 medium)
Pineapple	90 gm (5–6 thin round slices)
Coconut water	200 ml (1 glass)

Vegetable exchange

Group A

All green, leafy vegetables except those mentioned as Group B vegetables. They are negligible in calories.

Group B

100 gm = 1 exchange = 1 bowl provides carbohydrates 7 gm; proteins 2 gm; calories 36

Carrot	100 gm
Beetroot	100 gm
Green mango	100 gm
Beans	100 gm
Green pea	100 gm
Onion	100 gm
Lotus stem	100 gm

Root and tuber exchange
100 gm = 1 exchange = 1 bowl provides carbohydrates
25 gm; calories 100

Potato
Sweet potato
Yam
Colocasia
Tapioca

Note: Avoid roots and tubers or limit them to very small quantities because they yield high amounts of rapidly digestible carbohydrates and cause post-meal spikes in blood glucose.

Fat/oil exchange
Each exchange provides fat 5 gm; calories 45

Safflower	5 gm (1 tsp)
Sunflower	5 gm (1 tsp)
Soya	5 gm (1 tsp)
Mustard	5 gm (1 tsp)
Groundnut	5 gm (1 tsp)
Sesame	5 gm (1 tsp)
Vanaspati	5 gm (1 tsp)
Cream	10 gm (2 tsp)

BASIC HOUSEHOLD MEASURES

Ensure that your teaspoons, tablespoons and cups measure
up to the following universally accepted capacities:

1 teaspoon (tsp) = 5 ml
1 tablespoon (tbsp) = 15 ml
1 cup = 150 ml

Sample Meal Plan of 1800 Calories

Meal	Food Items
Morning snack	1 cup tea/coffee (with 50 ml milk)
Breakfast	2 small chapatis / 2 large bread slices / 2 medium idlis (avoid coconut chutney, replace with green chutney) + 1 cup cow's milk/1 egg + 1 tsp butter/oil/ghee
Mid-morning snack (mid-point between breakfast and lunch)	1 small apple/orange/sweet lime or ½ mango
Lunch	3 chapatis / 2 chapatis + 3 tbsp rice + 1½ small bowl dal + 100 ml curd + 1–2 small bowls green leafy vegetables + 1 small bowl Group B vegetables + 1 tsp oil for cooking
Afternoon tea	1 cup tea/coffee + 2 bread slices (avoid jam, replace with ½ tsp butter or green chutney)
Evening snack	1 small apple/orange/sweet lime or ½ mango
Dinner	Same as lunch
Bedtime snack	1 cup milk (without sugar) + 2 biscuits

Note: Non-vegetarians can replace curd at lunch/dinner with 30 gm mutton
or 50 gm chicken or 60 gm fish.

Sugar substitutes

Aspartame and sucralose are two very common sugar substitutes. They are reasonably safe and recommended for diabetics by many national diabetic associations including the ADA. These are available in various forms such as tablets, drops and powder. They do not have any calories whatsoever. Powdered sucralose was introduced in India in late 2005. Since it is heat-stable, it can be mixed with the raw material before it is subjected to high cooking temperature. With the known Indian fondness for sweets, the availability of sucralose is a boon for those who can now eat their favourite desserts like jalebis, rasgullas, cookies, cakes and pastries. Of course, you should eat desserts in very limited quantities, even if they don't contain sugar.

General guidelines

There are some foods that you must consume in very limited quantities. Here is a list to which you can keep adding as you get more information from other sources, especially your doctors and diabetologists.

- Fried snacks like chips, wafers, chivda (rice flakes), sev (fried flour noodles), papad (poppadums), bhajia (fritters)
- Saturated fats like butter, cream, ghee, animal fat, fatty meat (beef, lamb, pork, ham, organ meat), coconut oil, vanaspati
- Foods rich in cholesterol like egg yolk and organ meat (brain, liver)

- Nuts and oilseeds like cashew nut, pistachio, walnut, groundnut, coconut
- Beer, wines, whisky and other alcoholic drinks. (In fact, these are best avoided. If you cannot abstain, cut down on your intake drastically and calculate the calories provided by alcohol in your meal plan. Remember, 1 gm of alcohol gives 7 calories.)
- High-salt foods like papad, pickles, coconut chutney, most processed/preserved foods, dried fish, cured meat and foods containing baking soda and baking powder. (Excess salt raises your blood pressure. Diabetes and high blood pressure are independent risk factors for heart disease, and kidney and eye damage. When they are present together, the risk is not merely added up but compounded. And mind you, there is no difference in the chemical composition of rock salt and common salt, so don't be misled by the popular misconception that rock salt is a healthy substitute for common salt. Your salt intake should not exceed 5 gm per day.)

And then there are foods that you should totally avoid, such as simple sugars like glucose, dextrose, common sugar, candy, honey, jaggery, jam, jelly, syrups, marmalade, cakes, pastries, pies, puddings, ice cream, sweet biscuits, sweetmeats, chocolates, condensed milk, aerated drinks, tinned juices and sweet/oily pickles.

CEREAL KILLERS!

The market is flooded with several attractively packaged, branded, ready-to-eat cereal preparations. These contain various cereals in flaked form, usually fortified with vitamins and minerals. Remember that if you consume a balanced diet at home, you do not require these extra vitamins and minerals. However, aggressive advertising can misguide consumers and many families with average incomes may end up spending heavily on these products, which are several times costlier than home-made, freshly prepared, cereal-based dishes such as poha, upma, idli, and dosa. What is more, these branded products invariably contain high sugar and high salt, which are not recommended.

A Few Meal Planning Tools

Glycaemic index

The glycaemic index (GI) helps you rank carbohydrate-containing foods as per their potential to raise blood glucose compared with an equivalent amount of glucose. Pure glucose obviously has the highest GI of 100. To calculate the GI of a food, the rise in blood glucose over a period of two hours following the ingestion of 50 gm of the food being tested is compared with the rise in blood glucose following the ingestion of 50 gm of pure glucose. Over 600 food items have been assigned GI values.

In general, foods that break down quickly have higher GI values compared with those that break down and get digested slowly. So, a naan made of maida has a higher GI than a chapati made with wholewheat atta.

The GI value of a food also depends on the amount of viscous fibre it contains: the more the fibre, the lower the GI, which is why beans have a lower GI than potatoes. Other factors include the amount of fat present. At times, the decision can be tough! For instance, French fries have a lower GI compared with mashed potato. So, based on GI, they are a better choice than mashed potato because they raise blood glucose to a lesser extent than the same amount of mashed potato. Yet they provide more calories and cause weight gain because of their fat content, thus nullifying the advantage.

GI values also depend on several other variables including degree of ripeness (in the case of fruit), method of cooking, amount of water and other liquids consumed during a meal, and amount of fat eaten along with a carbohydrate-containing dish.

Some high GI foods are mashed potato, ripe banana, honey and maida-based preparations; medium GI foods are French fries, rice and chapatti); low GI foods are chana dal, brown rice and chapatis made of gram flour. For a longer list, see the table on the next page.

Glycaemic Index (GI) Values of Some Common Foods

Food	GI
Glucose	100
Mashed potato	80–90
Honey	80–90
Cornflakes	80–89
Rice	70–79
Brown bread/chapati	70–79
Upma	70–79
Banana	60–69
Beetroot	60–69
Potato chips	50–59
Idli	50–59
Yam	50–59
Orange	40–49
Black gram (urad dal)	40–49
Raw banana	40–49
Orange juice	40–49
Green gram (mung dal)	40–49
Ice cream	40–49
Bengal gram (chana dal)	30–39
Orange	30–39
Curd	30–39
Whole milk	30–39
Apple	30–39
Kidney beans (rajma)	20–29
Tomato	10–19
Green vegetables	10–19

Note: For the complete list, log on to www.diabetes.org

While planning your meals and exchanges, select foods with low GI to minimize post-prandial rise in blood glucose level. Do note, for instance, that fatty food has lower GI compared with food with lower fat content (potato chips versus mashed potato), so do not depend on GI as the sole factor for making food choices. This index helps you to select an item from the same food category, so you can go for oranges over bananas, upma over cornflakes and so on.

Carbohydrate counting and carbohydrate–insulin ratio

Carbohydrate counting (CC) is used most commonly in the US. The carbohydrate content of foods to be consumed during major meals and snacks is calculated from CC charts to decide the dosage of pre-meal insulin. Say you plan to have 3 chapatis, each weighing 20 gm—you will thus consume 45 gm of carbohydrates. If you also plan to have 1 bowl of mung dal and 2 bowls of green leafy vegetables, that will be another 25 gm of carbohydrates, so your total carbohydrate consumption from the meal would be 70 gm. If you are on insulin, you can work out your insulin dose based on this information. On average, one requires 1 unit of insulin for 15 gm of carbohydrates so your pre-meal insulin dose for this meal would be 5 units. If you plan to eat a little more or a little less, or if you plan to eat a different food item for your next meal, you can calculate your carbohydrates and adjust your insulin dose accordingly. Thus the CC method offers you flexibility in your food intake.

Please note that the carbohydrate-to-insulin ratio varies from person to person, depending on sensitivity to insulin. Some require 1 unit of insulin for each 10 gm of carbohydrates while others require 1 unit for each 12 gm of carbohydrates. However, one can initiate insulin therapy with the 1 unit per 15 gm carbohydrates formula, monitor post-meal blood glucose and then fine-tune or 'titrate' insulin dosage as per requirement.

It is mandatory for food manufacturers to declare the food contents per serving size as well as units in grams on the package. The information includes the amount of carbohydrates. For foods without labels, make an estimate, keeping the general serving size in mind. The following food items provide about 15 gm of carbohydrates:

- 1 small fresh fruit
- 1 large bread slice
- 1 small chapati
- 1/3 cup rice
- ½ cup oatmeal
- ½ cup black beans or starchy vegetables

EATING OUT

These days, you cannot avoid eating out, be it for social or professional purposes. The good news is that a diabetic need not shun this activity—he simply needs to be smart about it. When one eats out, despite careful planning and ordering, one eats food that is different from what one usually eats at home (in terms of ingredients, cooking medium, spices and so on). This is likely to adversely affect blood glucose level. To minimize these adverse effects, remember the following:

Frequency: Control how many times you eat out. Eat out only once a week. After a while, when you have well-controlled glucose levels and have mastered the art of food selection and portion sizes, you can eat out a little more frequently.

Timing: Stick to your schedule. If your usual dinner time is 9 p.m., then eat at 9 p.m., whether you are at a restaurant or at a party. If you cannot avoid eating later than that, eat a small snack at your usual time and reduce dinner appropriately.

Venue and food selection: If you can decide the venue, select a restaurant that offers a buffet with a large selection of salads and simply fill up your plate with those! If you are limited to à la carte service, order only after you ask pertinent questions about ingredients, cooking mediums, spices, portion sizes, etc. Order low-oil preparations, wholewheat breads and rotis, and broth-based clear soups. Avoid starters or have only starters, instead of the main course. Ask for salad dressings, butter, cream and sauces to be served on the side so that you can control your intake.

Choose broiled, baked, poached or grilled meats and fish over fried preparations. Avoid or minimize desserts, or have your fill of fruit. In a sit-down dinner, skip the dessert and have decaffeinated coffee.

Insulin injections: To avoid a dip in blood glucose, check on and anticipate the time it will take for the food to reach you after you place your order (in a restaurant). Accordingly, plan when to inject your insulin. If you are on rapid-acting insulin analogues or pre-mixed insulin containing rapid-acting insulin analogues, you can inject it after the food arrives at your table.

Monitoring the effects: Check your blood glucose levels two hours after eating out and compare them with your usual values after regular home food at that time. Correlate the blood glucose level with the type and amount of food you ate and use this information to optimize your next eat-out. For instance, let's say you could not resist the plate of dessert and your post-prandial blood glucose rose to 258 mg%. Well, the next time, simply avoid the dessert and then cross-check the values.

MANAGING DIABETES: PHYSICAL EXERCISE

Your meal plan, medication regimen, exercise schedule and knowledge of diabetes in all its aspects form the four cornerstones in the management of diabetes. However, exercise is usually the most neglected corner! If a diabetic is mindful of exercising properly and regularly, he can benefit immensely.

Benefits of Exercise

- Improves metabolic control (better control of blood glucose)
- Helps reduce dosage of insulin and oral drugs
- Catalyses weight reduction
- Along with diet control, helps control blood glucose level in many mild type 2 diabetics, thus pre-empting drug treatment
- Lowers blood pressure, commonly elevated in diabetics
- Helps reduce blood level of very low-density lipoprotein and low-density lipoprotein cholesterol (harmful fractions of blood fat, which if elevated cause serious problems like heart attacks) and helps increase blood level of high-

density lipoprotein cholesterol (protective fraction of blood fat)

- Improves blood circulation in the legs (many long-term diabetics suffer from poor blood circulation in the legs)
- Augments physical fitness and stamina
- Imparts a sense of well-being and improves psychological status

Precautions Before You Start Exercising

Inappropriate exercise can be hazardous, so always consult your doctor to plan your exercise schedule and intensity. He will first carry out a detailed physical examination and certain laboratory investigations (including an electrocardiogram) to ensure the following:

Good control of blood glucose level

Starting vigorous exercise in poorly controlled diabetics could worsen blood glucose control and precipitate an emergency. When you exercise, the body needs energy, which comes from the burning of glucose in the cells. Now, this glucose can enter your cells only with the help of insulin. If you have severe insulin deficiency, the glucose cannot enter the cell and will accumulate in the blood, making blood glucose levels spiral out of control.

Stability of cardiovascular system

Ischaemic heart disease is more common in diabetics and can stay undetected if it has atypical symptoms. Sudden vigorous exercise could precipitate serious problems such as a heart attack.

Absence of proliferative retinopathy

Long-term, poorly controlled diabetics usually have this complication. If they indulge in sudden vigorous exercise, such as jumping, they can suffer from vitreous haemorrhage, which can further reduce the vision. It is very important for long-term diabetics and diabetics with diminished vision to undergo a fundoscopy (inner eye examination) before they embark on any exercise.

Prevention of hypoglycaemia

Your doctor will also advise you on the proper time to exercise, in relationship with the timings of your meals and medications as well as dosage adjustments. The ideal time to exercise is in the morning after a light snack to pre-empt hypoglycaemia.

How to Prevent Hypoglycaemia

Do not exercise during peak insulin time—around three hours after plain insulin (Actrapid, Huminsulin R) and around seven hours after intermediate insulin (Huminsulin N, NPH insulin).

Do not inject insulin in the exercising arm. Exercise hastens absorption of insulin and may precipitate hypoglycaemia.

Remember that hypoglycaemia may unexpectedly occur very late at night, even after morning exercise. Test your blood glucose at different hours with a glucometer so that you can take dietary supplements at proper times or adjust the dosage of drugs. Such elaborate monitoring is required only initially to study your individual response pattern.

Make sure that your feet are healthy and you do not have any open wounds.

Which Type of Exercise Is Ideal?

Exercises are basically either dynamic (aerobic) or static (anaerobic).

In dynamic exercises, the major muscle groups are stretched in a rhythmic pattern and the entire body is in motion. Some examples are walking, jogging, cycling and swimming. In static exercise, your muscles contract against fixed objects while the body is static. Some examples are pressing palms against the wall or lifting weights.

In dynamic exercise, a large amount of energy is spent gradually over a period of time, and it is ideal for diabetic patients. Depending on your age, sex, physical condition and cardiovascular status, you should select a dynamic exercise regimen in consultation with your doctor. See the figure on the facing page to calculate the approximate calories spent per minute while doing dynamic exercises.

Type of exercise	Calories spent/minute
1. Brisk walking	3.6
2. Cycling	4.5
3. Jogging	4.5
4. Running	5.0
5. Swimming	6.0
6. Tennis (singles)	7.0

If you are middle-aged or beyond, brisk walking is a safe, easy and inexpensive exercise option. All you have to do is invest in pair of well-fitting and comfortable walking shoes. Younger, fitter diabetics can choose from running, swimming, cycling, a game of tennis and so on. All these exercises are as beneficial as a workout in a gymnasium. Yoga, which is not really an exercise in its properly defined sense, does help you inculcate a sense of discipline, and is a beneficial complement to your regular dynamic exercise regimen.

How long?

Ideally, you should go in for 30–45 minutes of sustained dynamic exercise without a break. However, start with 10 minutes daily in the first week and gradually go up to 30–45 minutes daily over a month. Remember, sustained exercise is important. The exercise should be strenuous enough to raise your heartbeat to 75 per cent maximal heart rate for 10–15 minutes.

> To calculate your maximal heart rate (MHR), use this formula: MHR = 220 minus your age in years

If you have to occasionally skip your daily exercise, here is how you can compensate for it during the course of the day.

- Don't use the elevator—use the stairs instead.
- Park your vehicle far from your place of work—walk to work!
- If you use public transport, get down one stop earlier than usual, both to and from work.

How often?

If you want to derive real benefits, you must exercise at least five days a week.

Proper exercise is useful, safe, inexpensive and pleasant. An integral mode of management of diabetes, it should never be bypassed.

9

MANAGING DIABETES: MEDICATION REGIMEN

Doctors commonly prescribe oral anti-diabetics to reduce blood glucose in type 2 diabetics. These are very popular because of ease of administration as well as affordability of most pills. The pills currently available belong to the following classes of medicines.

Class I: Sulphonylureas

Four members of this class of medicines are freely available in India: glibenclamide (Daonil), glipizide (Glynase/Glide), gliclazide (Diamicron) and glimepiride (Amaryl/Zoryl). All have the same mechanism of action but differ in terms of onset and duration of action. They act by stimulating the beta cells in the pancreas to release insulin into the circulation. Hence, they are effective if the pancreas has some viable beta cells. Usually they are tolerated well but may produce a hypoglycaemic reaction if proper precautions are not followed. Shorter-acting agents such as glipizide and newer agents such as glimepiride are comparatively safer in the context of hypoglycaemic reactions. Longer-acting drugs such as glibenclamide are more potent and thus more likely to produce hypoglycaemia.

Along with diet control, exercise and metformin (drug of another class, discussed right after this), sulphonylureas are the mainstay of management in most type 2 diabetics. One of the sulphonylureas is usually added when diet, exercise and metformin are insufficient to normalize blood glucose levels. They are effective for varying periods. However, after a few years of use, many patients gradually respond less and less and require insulin.

In certain complicated situations, such as impaired kidney and liver function, these medicines should not be used: because the body eliminates them slowly in the presence of kidney and liver disease, they are more liable to produce hypoglycaemia. They should be temporarily replaced by insulin during stressful situations, such as severe infections (tuberculosis), medical emergencies (heart attack) and major surgery. They should also not be used during pregnancy and lactation.

Benefits

1. Easily available
2. Well known to doctors, having been in continuous use for about six decades
3. Usually tolerated well by patients
4. Least expensive among all anti-diabetics (along with metformin)

Limitations

1. Effective only if pancreas has viable beta cells
2. Cause weight gain
3. May cause hypoglycaemic reactions

Class II: Biguanides

Metformin (Glyciphage) is the only member of this family that is universally available. It reduces blood glucose not by stimulating beta cells to secrete more insulin, but by increasing tissue sensitivity to the body's own insulin. When used as the sole agent to control blood glucose, it is unlikely to cause a hypoglycaemic reaction. Moreover, metformin is weight-neutral, not likely to cause weight gain unlike insulin and sulphonylureas. In fact, some patients may notice a slight reduction in weight. This is a major advantage, considering that long-term weight gain in diabetics is directly linked with higher risk of heart complications.

Metformin is the drug of first choice in type 2 diabetics. Unless specifically contraindicated or not tolerated, it should be used as a first-line agent. It should be taken after food to avoid unpleasant symptoms such as nausea, vomiting and abdominal pain. Most manufacturers of metformin now also offer 'slow release' tablets, which release active metformin gradually, over a period of time, into the intestine.

At times, patients on 'slow release' metformin pass off what appear to be intact tablets in stools and fret that they have wasted their hard-earned money on these tablets and will still be vulnerable to complications. They need not worry: the active agent metformin is gradually released through the outer coating or shell and this shell devoid of any active ingredient may be egested along with faeces.

Diabetics who are pregnant or lactating or suffering from kidney or liver disease should not use metformin. Those on metformin should absolutely avoid alcohol, as alcohol intake may lead to life-threatening episodes of lactic acidosis.

Benefits of conventional biguanides

- Do not cause weight gain
- Unlikely to cause hypoglycaemia if used as sole agents
- May help bring down insulin dosage in some patients, if used judiciously

Benefits of slow-release biguanides

- Need to be administered less frequently
- Have fewer side effects such as diarrhoea and abdominal discomfort

Limitations

- In 5–10 per cent of the patients, metformin may cause nausea, vomiting and/or abdominal pain if taken on empty stomach

Class III: Non-sulphonylurea Secretagogues[1]

Repaglinide (Eurepa/Regan) is the first member of a new class of drugs that act somewhat like sulphonylureas but are structurally different. In their case, onset of action is much quicker than in sulphonylureas, and thus is specially suited to control post-meal rise in blood glucose. This drug is also relatively safe in that it is less likely to cause hypoglycaemic reactions and can be safe despite impaired kidney function. However, it needs to be given two to three times daily. Some manufacturers promote repaglinide aggressively for diabetics with irregular and undisciplined lifestyle, focusing on its relative safety as regards hypoglycaemia. Patients may think, therefore, that if they are on repaglinide, they need not be regular with their meal timings. This is a misconception though. Dietary control is an irreplaceable mode of diabetes management and also one of the factors that your doctor considers when prescribing your medicine dosage.

Nateglinide (Glinate), another drug in this class, was introduced some years ago. It has a slight edge over repaglinide because it is absorbed even quicker, though it has a slightly shorter duration of action. It is marginally better at controlling post-prandial rise in blood glucose and pre-empting hypoglycaemia.

---

1 A secretagogue is a substance that causes another substance (especially endocrine, exocrine or paracrine) to be secreted

Benefits

- More effective than sulphonylureas in controlling post-prandial blood glucose and avoiding hypoglycaemia

Limitations

- Costlier than sulphonylureas
- Less effective than sulphonylureas at controlling fasting blood glucose
- Need to be taken three times a day

Class IV: Glitazones

This relatively new class of agents, also known as thiazolindinediones, was introduced in India in the late 1990s. Two members of this class are rosiglitazone (Rezult/ Enselin) and pioglitazone (Pioglit).

Like biguanides, these agents are insulin sensitizers. They do not stimulate the release of insulin but increase the effectiveness of already available insulin—either the body's own or that administered via injections. They increase the sensitivity of your tissues towards insulin and thus get more out of the body's own insulin. Thus these agents are useful in diabetics who have insulin resistance.

The main sites of action of glitazones are muscles and fat tissues—compare this with metformin, which also corrects insulin resistance but acts mainly at the liver. Thus, the action of glitazones complements those of metformin and sulphonylureas, as well as insulin. They can be given as monotherapy to diabetics who have severe insulin resistance and cannot use metformin; in others, they can be combined with other anti-diabetic drugs for added advantages.

If you have a liver disease or heart failure (including past history) or if you are pregnant, you should not use glitazones. A patient who is prescribed a glitazone needs to be monitored for liver functions before starting therapy, and subsequently at two-monthly intervals. Some patients on glitazones gain significant weight, sometimes as much as 7–8 kg.

In 2007, it was observed that patients on rosiglitazone were a bit more likely to develop heart attack and die of sudden cardiac death compared with those on other anti-diabetic medications including pioglitazone, a member of the same glitazone family. Subsequent to this observation and after a lot of debate, the common use of rosiglitazone was banned globally in 2010. Recently pioglitazone use was linked with cancer of the urinary bladder. France and Germany have banned the common use of this medicine, while in other countries including the US, other European countries including the UK, and in India, pioglitazone is still freely available but is under close scrutiny of the respective drug regulatory authorities.

Benefits

- Unlikely to cause hypoglycaemia when used as sole agents
- Effective for longer than sulphonylureas and biguanides

Limitations

- Contraindicated in patients with liver disease, heart failure or pregnancy
- May cause significant weight gain in some patients

Class V: Alpha-Glucosidase Inhibitors

These agents, AGIs in short, were introduced in India in the late 1990s, starting with the prototype acarbose (Glucobay) and followed by miglitol (Mignar) and voglibose (Volibo). These agents act on the small intestine and slow down the process of digestion of carbohydrates, thus slowing down the rate of formation of glucose in the intestines and its absorption into the blood circulation. This helps reduce blood glucose peaks after meals. AGIs are thus specially suited to control post-meal blood glucose spiking.

For mild diabetics, they can be used as monotherapy. When used as monotherapy, they do not cause hypoglycaemia. For regular diabetics, they can be combined with other oral drugs or insulin. However, remember, when given along with insulin or sulphonylureas, they can cause hypoglycaemia.

The main difference between AGIs and other agents is that while AGIs act on the surface of the intestines, all other oral anti-diabetics act after they are absorbed into the bloodstream. Some patients on AGIs complain of gaseous distension of the abdomen, flatulence and diarrhoea.

Benefits

- Especially suitable for post-prandial control of blood glucose level
- Work in synergy with all other anti-diabetic agents

Limitations

- Cause side effects such as flatulence (socially embarrassing), abdominal distension and diarrhoea
- Have limited overall efficacy

Class VI: DPP4 Inhibitors (Gliptins)

These are the latest anti-diabetic pills. Sitagliptin (Januvia), the prototype of this class, was introduced in India around 2007, after which vildagliptin (Galvus), saxagliptin (Onglyza) and linagliptin (Tragenta) hit the markets in quick succession.

These agents act on the small intestine and raise the level of GLP1, a natural hormone. Type 2 diabetics have a deficiency of GLP1, which leads to deficiency of insulin and excessive post-prandial production of glucagon. Both abnormalities are responsible for high blood glucose levels. Gliptins correct both abnormalities and thus normalize the elevated blood glucose levels. They are immensely popular because they do not cause weight gain and also do not cause hypoglycaemia.

The availability of these agents has widened the choice of anti-diabetic agents and definitely led to better control of blood glucose in many patients. Many experts expect these to replace sulphonylureas in the future. However, they are five to ten times costlier than sulphonylureas and have been around only for about five years while sulphonylureas have been in continuous use for almost sixty years.

Benefits

- Are unlikely to cause hypoglycaemia when used as solo therapy or in sync with insulin sensitizers
- Do not cause weight gain
- Are likely to be protective for the heart (research under way)

Limitations

- Are expensive (five to ten times costlier than sulphonylureas)[2]

Class VII: Non-Insulin Anti-diabetic Injectables (Incretin Mimetics)

Two agents of this class are currently available: (1) exenatide and (2) liraglutide. Both are useful in type 2 diabetics. While

2 In end-March 2013, close on the heels of a landmark judgement by the Supreme Court of India concerning patents on medicines, the pharmaceutical manufacturer Glenmark introduced its brand of sitagliptin at 60 per cent of the price of MSD's version, branded as Januvia. MSD feels that Glenmark's action is illegal and has moved court seeking the withdrawal of Glenmark's brand from the market. Let us wait and watch. Diabetics will be the real winners if the court rules in favour of Glenmark.

the former needs to be injected twice a day, the latter needs to be administered once a day. Both are potent agents and have the inherent advantage of not causing hypoglycaemia clubbed with the ability to actually reduce weight. However, these are expensive (cost about Rs 8000 a month) and need to be injected instead of swallowed.

There is a slow-release version of exenatide, which needs to be injected only once a week. It has recently been introduced in some countries and should be available in India in the near future. As you can gather, these agents are suitable for you if you are a type 2 diabetic keen to lose weight and prepared to take expensive injections.

Benefits

- Do not cause hypoglycaemia
- Help reduce weight

Limitations

- Need to be injected (but are painless)
- Are expensive
- May not be easily available in non-urban areas

PILL POINTERS

Ten-Point Checklist on Medications That Lower Blood Sugar

1. Carefully follow the medicine dosage schedule prescribed by your doctor.
2. Carefully follow all aspects of dietary advice suggested by your diabetologist.
3. Remember that just because you are on anti-diabetic pills, it does not mean that you have the licence to eat any food in any amount.
4. Monitor your statistics by getting your blood glucose lab-tested every three months, your glycosylated haemoglobin every six months and your kidney function every year (unless impaired, in which case monitoring would be more frequent). Alongside, self-monitor your blood glucose with a glucometer. The frequency of monitoring will depend on several factors, including type of diabetes, insulin dependency, degree of control, tendency to hypoglycaemia and special situations (pregnancy).
5. If your blood glucose is well controlled, gradually reduce pill dosage on your doctor's advice.
6. If blood glucose values are persistently high despite gradually increasing pill dosage till the highest level, there is no point persisting with the pills. Accept the

doctor's advice and start on insulin. With modern superfine needles, injections are practically painless, so don't pressurize your doctor to continue prescribing pills.

7. If your kidney or liver functions are impaired, you may suffer from complications such as hypoglycaemia due to slow elimination of pills from your system. In such a case, change over to insulin on your doctor's advice.

8. Avoid alcohol as far as possible.

9. Be aware of and smart about drug interactions. When a patient is prescribed two medicines, they may affect each other's actions, by either dominating or diminishing. Many diabetics also suffer from other diseases like high blood pressure and heart disorders, so they are likely to take several medicines together. Always share details of your current treatment with your doctors. The following drugs enhance the blood glucose lowering effect of sulphonylureas: Dicumarol (anticoagulant prescribed to some heart patients), Monoamine Oxidase inhibitors (antidepressants) and common painkillers. If you take any of them, the dosage of your anti-diabetic may need to be scaled down. On the other hand, if you need corticosteroids, you may need to increase dosage or even shift to insulin for some time.

10. Do not stay hungry for long periods, and definitely do not fast. Eat small but frequent meals.

10

HOW DOES INSULIN HELP MANAGE DIABETES?

Insulin is an important hormone formed in the pancreas, an endocrine gland situated in the abdomen behind the stomach. An important dual-purpose gland, the pancreas produces not only various hormones (including insulin) but also digestive enzymes. The hormones are formed in islands of specialized cells called islets of Langerhans. The insulin-making cells situated in these islands are known as beta cells.

Insulin is an important hormone involved in metabolism. It facilitates the entry of glucose into tissues and inhibits the formation of glucose in the liver, thus helping maintain blood glucose levels in the normal range. In diabetics, there is a deficiency of insulin, either absolute or relative, and that causes a rise in blood glucose level.

In normal people, who do not suffer from a diabetic condition, insulin formation is automatically controlled. After food intake—which is when carbohydrates are digested and converted into glucose—more insulin is formed and released to control the rise in blood glucose level. In a fasting state, insulin formation/release is suppressed. This is how blood glucose is always maintained in the normal range in normal people.

How Does Insulin Control Blood Glucose?

Insulin plays a dual role while controlling blood glucose levels. It facilitates the entry of glucose into tissue cells. In other words, it opens the door of muscle cells and lets glucose enter the cells. Once inside, glucose is either burnt to release energy or converted into glycogen and stored. Insulin's action on the cells is mediated through its interaction with insulin receptors situated on the cell surface. Thus insulin and its specific receptor act as a key and a lock respectively. Their interaction leads to the opening of doors of muscle cells and entry of glucose into the cells. The other important site of action of insulin is the liver. Here it suppresses the formation of glucose by inhibiting gluconeogenesis (formation of glucose from proteins) and glycogenolysis (conversion of glycogen

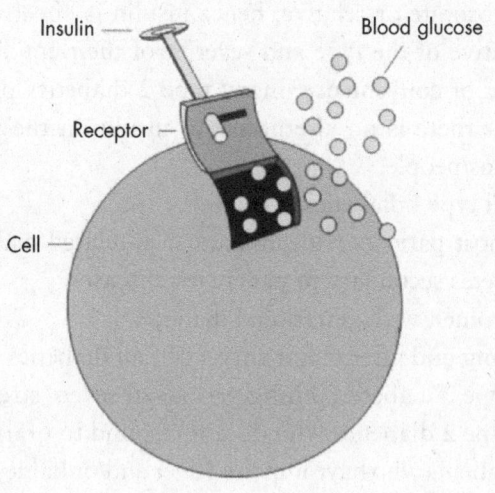

into glucose). In a fasting state, the liver is the main source of glucose; in a fed state, carbohydrates from food are the main source. In a severe diabetic state, blood glucose remains persistently high even if the patient hardly takes anything by mouth, because in the absence of adequate insulin, the liver produces a large amount of glucose and releases it into the bloodstream.

Who Needs Insulin?

Being a protein, insulin is split into individual amino acids if ingested by mouth. Hence it is ineffective when given by mouth. It has to be injected, usually subcutaneously (into the layer of fat that lies just below the skin), from where it is absorbed whole into the circulation and carried to the site of action. In diabetics, there is a deficiency of insulin, either absolute or relative, hence insulin is effective for all, irrespective of the type and severity of their condition. For the sake of convenience, many type 2 diabetics prefer oral pills but there is no alternative to insulin in the following situations/people:

1. In all type I diabetics
2. In most patients with malnutrition-related diabetes and diabetes secondary to pancreatic diseases
3. In women with gestational diabetes
4. During and after major surgery in all diabetics
5. In type 2 diabetics during periods of severe stress
6. In type 2 diabetics who do not respond to oral pills
7. In patients who have impaired liver and/or kidney function

HISTORY OF INSULIN

The introduction of insulin in 1921-22 was one of the greatest milestones in medical research. It revolutionized the use of the body's own proteins as a medication. Till insulin was introduced into daily practice, the diagnosis of type 1 diabetes—then called juvenile diabetes—meant certain death within months, maybe even weeks.

Insulin was first isolated in the laboratories of the University of Toronto in Canada. Dr Fredrick Banting, Charlie Best (a medical student at the time), Prof. J. MacLeod and Dr James Collip were jointly given credit for this discovery.

The very first patient to receive an insulin injection for the treatment of diabetes was Leonard Thomson (1908–1935). Leonard was terminally ill when he was injected on 11 January 1922. Soon after he started the treatment, he made a rapid recovery and went on to live for another thirteen years.

The insulin injection that Leonard received then and the various types of insulin used today are poles apart. The first insulin was a crude extract from ox pancreas while today's insulin is highly purified human insulin manufactured by genetic engineering technology. Between these two poles and over ninety years, several milestones have been crossed. The availability of increasingly better and more effective insulin to manage diabetes is due to continuous evolution and painstaking research. In fact, some exciting new types of insulin (those that act even quicker and those that are efficacious for longer than existing ones) are being developed as you read, and will soon be available to make life easier for diabetics.

How Many Types of Insulin Are There?

Depending on its structure, purity and speed of action, insulin is classified in the following various ways.

Structure-based insulin types

Bovine insulin

This is prepared by extraction from the pancreas of a cow or bull. Till the turn of the twenty-first century, bovine insulin was the cheapest in the market and was extensively used in India. Except in patients allergic to it or pregnant diabetics or those who required extremely large doses due to partial neutralization by insulin antibody formation, bovine insulin was almost as good as human insulin. Now that the cost difference between bovine and human insulin is negligible, bovine insulin has almost been phased out.

Porcine insulin

This is prepared by extraction from the pancreas of a pig. Structurally, it is nearer to human insulin than bovine insulin, so fewer patients are allergic to it. The gradual increase in its cost and simultaneous reduction in the cost of human insulin has made porcine insulin nearly disappear from the market.

Human insulin

Structurally, it resembles the insulin formed in our pancreas exactly. It is manufactured either by a semi-synthetic process (porcine insulin is purified and converted into human insulin) or a bio-synthetic process (using genetic engineering techniques). Manufacturers have gradually transitioned to the bio-synthetic process, virtually eliminating raw material shortage and preventing cost escalations.

Purity-based insulin types

Conventional insulin

This contains small quantities of other pancreatic proteins in addition to insulin. It was earlier called 'impure insulin'. Bovine insulin available in India belonged to this class until recently. Manufacturers of bovine insulin have upgraded their process of purification recently, so currently marketed bovine insulin is almost as pure as human insulin.

Highly purified and mono-component insulin

This is purified by chromatographic methods and hardly contains any non-insulin substances. Human insulin in India belongs to this class.

Speed-based insulin types

Short-acting insulin

Also known as crystalline insulin or plain insulin, it appears as a clear, watery solution. It is relatively rapidly absorbed from the site of injection. The action starts about thirty minutes after injection, peaks after two to three hours and extends for up to six hours. This is used to control post-meal rise in blood glucose. Some popular brands are Actrapid, Huminsulin-R and Lupisulin-R. It is often combined with intermediate-acting insulin.

Rapid-acting insulin

In some patients, short-acting insulin is not quick enough to control post-meal rise in blood glucose, so they need rapid-acting insulin. It has a quicker onset (within fifteen minutes) and shorter duration (90–120 minutes) of action. It is made by slightly altering the structure of natural insulin. Lispro, Apidra and Novorapid are some available brands. Since each manufacturer develops its own technology, rapid-acting insulin is also called designer's insulin or insulin analogue. Being more expensive than conventional insulin, it is used in special situations.

Intermediate-acting insulin

It is gradually absorbed from the site of injection so the onset of action is slower and the duration of action longer. Usually, onset is after two to three hours, peak action at around seven hours and duration of action around sixteen hours.

It is used to control fasting blood glucose. Insulatard and Huminsulin-N are some brands. It is cloudy in appearance.

Long-acting insulin (glargine)

Its duration of action is almost twenty-four hours; hence, it is given once a day, thus clearly scoring over intermediate-acting insulin which needs to be administered twice a day, particularly in type 1 diabetics. Moreover, the prevalence of hypoglycaemia with glargine (Lantus) is lower than with intermediate-acting insulin. It was launched in India in 2003 and has become extremely popular very rapidly. In 2006, detemir insulin (Levemir), another long-acting insulin with smooth, predictable action was introduced in India. Its price is close to that of glargine. In glargine as well as in detemir, the duration of action is prolonged by altering the structure of natural insulin. With each manufacturer inventing its own technology, these are also classified as insulin analogues or designer insulins.

Pre-mixed insulin

Short- and intermediate-acting insulin are pre-mixed in fixed proportion during the manufacturing process to simplify administration. Currently, this insulin is available in three variants (25/75, 30/70, 50/50), and in both conventional and analogue forms. Since it is cumbersome to mix shorter- and longer-acting insulin before administration, pre-mixed insulin is very popular, particularly in India where more than 80 per cent of insulin sold is a variant of pre-mixed insulin. On the flip side, this does not have the flexibility of free adjustment of proportion of two types of insulin. An experienced diabetologist decides when to prescribe pre-mixed insulin and when shorter- and longer-acting insulin separately. If precision is a must, he prescribes individual preparations to be mixed manually before injecting. If precision is not as vital as pragmatism, pre-mixed insulin is given.

FUTURE OF ANIMAL INSULIN

Around the mid-1980s, when highly purified porcine and human insulin were introduced in India, the prices were Rs 140 and Rs 210 rupees, respectively, for a vial of 400 units. Bovine insulin was then available for Rs 40 per vial. Naturally, in the initial years, fewer people used the newer insulin forms. Over the last two decades, the situation has changed. With the cost of human insulin gradually declining and that of bovine insulin gradually rising, there is barely any cost differential. Since human insulin is genetically engineered, raw material shortage is eliminated and costs cut drastically. Till recently, insulin was not manufactured in India. A few years ago, three Indian companies started manufacturing and selling human insulin, for the local and export market. This has brought down the price of some brands of human insulin to as low as Rs 130 per vial— lower than the price of animal insulin. Bovine insulin is thus likely to make an exit from the market. Major manufacturers of porcine insulin have already withdrawn their products and replaced them with human insulin brands. In any scenario, the diabetic patient is the clear winner.

Which Insulin Should I Take?

Once it is decided that you need insulin, your diabetologist will decide the type, frequency and quantity of insulin you need. Most type 1 diabetics, pancreatic diabetics and severely insulin-dependent type 2 diabetics need insulin at least twice a day. Usually, they are given a combination of short- and intermediate-acting insulin before breakfast and dinner. Short-acting insulin before breakfast helps control post-breakfast and post-lunch rise in blood glucose. By the time its action starts fading, intermediate-acting insulin takes over and keeps blood glucose under control till dinner. Similarly, short-acting insulin before dinner takes care of post-dinner rise in blood glucose and acts till about midnight when intermediate-acting insulin takes over and controls blood glucose through the night till the morning dose, and so on. Once exact individual needs are worked out, some patients can change over to appropriate pre-mixed insulin for convenience. Severe diabetics may need an additional shot of short-acting insulin before lunch, while those who started out as type 2 diabetics and retain some ability to form insulin in their pancreas can be controlled with only one shot of insulin, usually in addition to oral pills. In some cases, the evening dose of intermediate- or long-acting insulin is given at bedtime.

When Should I Inject Insulin?

Short-acting insulin (Actrapid, Huminsulin-R, Lupisulin-R) or pre-mixed insulin containing short-acting insulin (Mixtard 30/70, Mixtard 50/50, Huminsulin 30/70, Huminsulin 50/50, Lupisulin 30/70) should be injected thirty minutes before a meal. Rapid-acting insulin (Novorapid, Humalog, Apidra) or pre-mixed insulin containing it (Novomix, Humalog 25, Humalog 50) should be injected between ten minutes before eating to ten minutes after having eaten. Lantus and Levemir can be injected any time of the day, same time every day, irrespective of food timing.

DEVICES TO INJECT INSULIN

Syringes: Most diabetics prefer specially designed plastic syringes with fixed needles of very fine (no. 31) bore to make the process virtually painless. These syringes are disposable. However, even though manufacturers recommend single use, these can be safely used four to six times for the same patient, provided they are stored in absolutely hygienic conditions.

Refillable pens: Slightly longer and thicker than ordinary pens, these have insulin cartridges loaded within, and disposable needles attached at the lower end. You can set the desired insulin dose by rotating the upper part. After that, a simple click delivers the dose. The pen's advantages are that you can bypass the process of filling the syringe by withdrawing from a vial and that it delivers the precise dose of insulin, no more and no less. It is very simple to refill the pen with a new cartridge. The pen is ideal for those prepared to pay a little extra for convenience. Almost all insulin brands are now available in pens as well as vials. These pens are being improved gradually, and modern versions have facilities to reset the dose without discarding the insulin that has already been set, to set odd-unit doses, and to administer easily with a light push.

Disposable pens: All major insulin manufacturers have also launched disposable pen devices for their insulin. Each pen holds 300 units of insulin, after using up which you must discard the pen and get a new one. They are suitable for initiation of insulin treatment.

Jet injectors: The jet injector delivers insulin through multiple punctures. Like the pen, it offers the advantages of hiding the needle and hence is more acceptable than a syringe to some patients. However, it is very expensive— approximately Rs 25,000 per piece.

Insulin Vials or Pens: Which and When?

The traditional method of injecting insulin is to use a disposable plastic syringe to draw insulin from a glass vial, and inject it into the patient's body. It is the cheapest way but more cumbersome compared with using insulin pens. So if economy is your priority, use syringes and vials.

If you require more than 40 units of insulin at a time, you should use U/100 insulin vials and syringes to avoid an extra prick. (The capacity of a U/40 syringe is 40 units.) Another advantage of using insulin from a U/100 vial (with 100 as opposed to 40 units per ml) is that the reduced volume of injected insulin is less painful.

Insulin pens are quicker and smarter. What is more, the dosage they deliver is precise. The pen's upper portion is rotated clockwise till the numerical figure of insulin dose appears in a window at its upper end. This is known as 'dialling the dose'. Disposable pens are preloaded with an insulin cartridge within a sealed compartment. Once all the insulin (300 units) is used up, they cannot be refilled and must be discarded. In reusable pens, you need to insert an insulin cartridge refill every time you run through 300 units; it is as simple as replacing a ballpoint pen refill! If you are going to use insulin over a short term, or if you want to try out the suitability of pens, then use disposable pens. If you are a long-term user, go in for reusable pens, as they are more economical than disposables.

The cost of one unit of human insulin injected through syringe, reusable pen and disposable pen is 35 paise, 65 paise and 90 paise, respectively. The maximum one-time cost of a reusable pen is about a thousand rupees. Insulin analogues are usually available only in pens, with the exception of Lantus, which is also available in vials. If you drive a hard bargain, you could get yourself a reusable insulin pen free of cost—insulin in cartridge form has better profit margins, so companies can afford to give away free reusable pens, hoping that the patient will use them (and thus their insulin cartridges) for a long time.

BE ALERT WHEN USING VIALS AND SYRINGES!

In western countries, insulin is available in concentrated form, which is 100 units per ml (U/100). In India, even though U/100 insulin is available, more often than not U/40 insulin, containing 40 units per ml, is prescribed. Now, if you make the mistake of using U/100 insulin with syringes made for U/40 insulin, you will end up injecting 2.5 times the usual dose, thus leading to severe hypoglycaemia. On the other hand, if you happen to have some imported syringes meant for U/100 insulin and use those to inject U/40 insulin, you will take only 40 per cent of the usual dose, thus leading to hyperglycaemia. Always, always verify that the vial's insulin strength and the insulin syringe are compatible. By convention, U/100 syringes have orange caps while U/40 syringes have red caps. In contrast, pens have insulin only in U/100 strength and deliver insulin units directly so there is no risk of any such mismatch.

Mismatch between Vial and Syringe: A Grave Oversight

In India, the most popular way to administer insulin is subcutaneously, using a syringe. After prescribing insulin injections, it is the doctor's duty to ensure that the patient understands all the details, such as units and type of insulin, frequency of injection, time gap between injection and food intake, vial strength and specifications of insulin syringe.

Insulin vials are available in two strengths: U/40 containing 40 units per ml and U/100 containing 100 units per ml. Insulin syringes are also available in two types, U/40 and U/100, each made specifically to suit the corresponding vial. Besides teaching the proper injection technique, the treating doctor must brief the patient about different vial strengths and syringe types. He should advise the patient to always verify the vial strength whenever he uses a new vial and to always withdraw insulin in matching syringes.

However, major mistakes do occur, due to carelessness on the part of the doctor or the patient. These mistakes can lead to hypoglycaemia or hyperglycaemia and also create life-threatening emergencies. Here are a few case studies of such mistakes that I have come across.

Case 1: Doctor's error

A patient was on Inj. Huminsulin (30/70), U/40 vial, 40 units twice a day. Since his blood glucose was poorly controlled, he was advised Inj. Huminsulin (30/70), 50 units twice a day.

Since the capacity of a U/40 syringe is only 40 units, he was advised to use U/100 syringe so that he could avoid two pricks by taking insulin once up to the 50-units mark. The patient followed the advice but his blood glucose level worsened. The reason was obvious. If one takes U/40 insulin up to the 50-unit mark in a U/100 syringe, he actually takes only 20 units. So, instead of increasing the insulin from 40 units to 50 units, he ended up reducing it to 20 units.

Take-home message
In such a situation, the doctor should have advised the patient to change over to U/100 vial paired with U/100 syringe or to simply make the transition to insulin pens.

Case 2: Illiterate patient

An uneducated patient was on Inj. Mixtard (30/70), 48 units before breakfast and 34 units before dinner. His blood glucose was very high though his compliance with insulin injections as well as his diet control was flawless. During investigations, he could not answer questions about the syringe specification but he did know the cost of his insulin vial, so we could deduce that he was on U/40 insulin. (To find out the strength of insulin vial in the case of uneducated patients, we check on vial cost. A U/40 vial costs 125–150 rupees while a U/100 vial costs over 300 rupees.) Then we found that his vial lasted two and a half times the expected period. We figured that he was taking U/40 insulin via U/100 syringe, thus actually taking only 40 per cent of the prescribed dose. We asked him to bring his vial and syringe, and the inference was confirmed. He changed over to U/40 syringe and soon his blood glucose was well controlled.

Take-home message

If your blood glucose is erratic despite your adhering to medication and diet plans, find out how many days the vial lasts. If it lasts much longer than expected, there could be a mismatch between vial and syringe.

It is quite likely that you are injecting insulin from a U/40 vial but with a U/100 syringe. So, if you are prescribed 20 units of insulin twice a day, you should finish the vial in 10 days. (Each vial contains 400 units of insulin, 40 units per ml in a 10 ml vial.) But if you use a U/100 syringe and draw insulin up to the 20-unit mark, you will end up using only 8 units of insulin at a time, or 16 units per day, so the vial will last for 25 days!

This error has a reason. Many Indian diabetics have relatives overseas. When these relatives discover that their Indian cousin needs insulin injections, they send large cartons of disposable insulin syringes. Now, these are invariably U/100 syringes, meant to inject U/100 insulin, the only strength available for common use in the entire developed world. In India, however, most patients use U/40 insulin. If insulin from U/40 vials is drawn up in U/100 syringes, patients end up injecting only 40 per cent of the prescribed dose (unless they draw 2.5 times the prescribed dose). So it is better to avoid using U/100 syringes for U/40 insulin. However, in an emergency, one may multiply the prescribed dose 2.5 times and use a U/100 syringe for U/40 insulin. For example, if one is prescribed 20 units of insulin and has a U/40 vial but a U/100 syringe, he should withdraw insulin from the U/40 vial till the 50-unit mark on the U/100 syringe.

On the other hand, in the extremely rare situation of having to inject U/100 insulin with a U/40 syringe, one has to multiply by a factor of 0.4. For example, if one is prescribed 20 units of insulin and has to draw that from a U/100 vial with a U/40 syringe, he should withdraw insulin up to the 8-unit mark on the U/40 syringe.

U/40 syringes have red caps and are marked up to 40, while U/100 syringes have orange caps and are marked up to 100.

Case 3: Being impractical

A patient was on Huminsulin (30/70), 40 units in the morning and 20 units in the evening. His fasting blood glucose was well controlled but his post-lunch level was high. So, his morning dose was increased to 44 units while the evening dose was unchanged. Since one can only take up to 40 units of insulin in a U/40 syringe, he was rightly advised to change over to a U/100 insulin vial and inject it with a U/100 insulin syringe. However, he continued to take his evening dose of 20 units from a U/40 vial with a U/40 syringe and ordered fresh stocks of U/40 vials and syringes even after the vial in use was finished.

He did not make any technical mistake but after using all the remaining insulin from a U/40 vial for the evening dose, he could have taken 20 units in the evening from the U/100 vial he used for the morning. There was no need to keep an inventory of two vial types and two syringe types!

Take-home message

You can use U/100 vials and syringes for small as well as large doses though you cannot inject more than 40 units of U/40 insulin with a U/40 syringe.

Case 4: Awareness lacunae

A patient was prescribed Huminsulin (30/70), U/40 vial, 10 units before dinner. She was doing well with appropriate syringes and vials purchased from the market till she received a vial of Huminsulin 30/70, U/100 free of cost from her employer's medical services department. Nobody briefed her about the difference between U/40 and U/100 vials and the need to use appropriate needles. For some days, she used U/40 syringes to inject insulin from U/100 vials. One fine day, her family doctor noticed the discrepancy between insulin and syringe. He decided to draw up to the 25-unit mark to account for the difference. In fact, he should have drawn up to the 4-unit mark. Thus, he injected 62.5 units and magnified the mistake further two and a half times. The patient developed severe hypoglycaemia.

Take-home message

All patients, caregivers and paramedics should receive intensive education on the different strengths of insulin vials and syringes. As far as possible, same-strength syringes and vials should be used. To avoid calculation mistakes, simply change over to insulin pens.

Case 5: Cost-cutting

A forty-three-year-old woman was prescribed Inj. Mixtard (30/70), 20 units before breakfast and dinner. Her blood glucose was stable till she decided to cut costs. She purchased U/40 vials of Mixtard (30/70) and used a syringe to draw insulin from it to refill her empty Mixtard cartridges. Soon her blood glucose skyrocketed. The reason is obvious. While the Mixtard cartridge contains U/100 insulin, Mixtard U/40 from a vial contains 40 units per ml. She ended up taking only 8 units of insulin twice a day instead of 20 units twice a day.

Take-home message

Thoughtless improvisation can be dangerous.

Case 6: Callous chemist

A sixty-six-year-old woman was prescribed Mixtard (30/70), 15 units before breakfast. She bought the vials and syringes from a chemist shop in a bylane. The chemist gave her U/100 vials but U/40 syringes. She regularly took 15 units of insulin daily before breakfast and experienced hypoglycaemic episodes now and then. When she came to us for a second opinion, we checked her vials and syringes and identified the mistake. We trained her to change over to U/40 vials and draw 15 units in U/40 syringes. We also briefed her daughter thoroughly.

Take-home message
Do not take anything for granted. Each time you make a fresh purchase of syringes and/or vials, physically inspect them to confirm compatibility.

Case 7: Blessing in disguise

A forty-three-year-old man, known diabetic for three years, was hospitalized following a heart attack. He was on intravenous insulin infusion for forty-eight hours and subsequently discharged on Mixtard (U/40), 10 units before breakfast and before dinner. When he came for follow-up after six weeks, his fasting and post-lunch plasma glucose values were 100 mg% and 132 mg%, respectively. Everything seemed okay but on routine verification, we found that his vials lasted much longer than expected. On further investigation, we found out that he was using a U/100 syringe to inject U/40 insulin so he was taking only 4 units of insulin twice a day. Yet, miraculously, his blood glucose was well controlled. We discontinued his insulin and kept him on aggressive lifestyle restrictions. When he came for a follow-up after four weeks, his fasting and post-lunch plasma glucose values were 96 mg% and 130 mg%, respectively. Had he taken the insulin as advised, he would have had hypoglycaemia. His insulin requirement probably dipped faster than anticipated due to disappearance of transient insulin resistance associated with a condition such as a heart attack.

Take-home message
Even if you are apparently doing well, don't take things for granted. Always verify compatibility between vials and syringes.

11

MONITORING
PROGRESS

Any project requires conscientious monitoring to ensure that it is on track, to detect early derailment, if any, and take immediate remedial action to put it back on track. Think of your diabetes management plan as just such a project. All pre-diabetics and diabetics, whether newly diagnosed or long-standing, should monitor their status very regularly and very mindfully. As they say, 'a stitch in time saves nine'. A small investment made in terms of time and money towards regular monitoring will go a long way in preventing very major expenses later, in terms of time (prolonged hospitalization) and associated monetary expenses.

It is shocking to find out that very few diabetics are careful enough to carry out periodic monitoring. As long as they feel all right and do not have symptoms of any complications, they continue their medication in dosages prescribed by their doctors years ago. They forget to take into account the fact that as their bodies, lifestyles and priorities change, so do their physical parameters, including blood pressure level and blood glucose level. And then, having been careless for way too long, some patients get hospitalized as emergency cases with complications such as hypoglycaemic coma or severe infections such as carbuncle or diabetic foot abscess or tuberculosis (linked to very high blood glucose levels).

You should always bear in mind that in a vibrant human body, nothing is constant and the need for anti-diabetic medicines also changes with time, depending on several factors and their interactions. Here are some examples:

If you get a little slack in your diet control and/or physical exercise regimen, your blood glucose values will shoot up. Then, if you suddenly clamp down on your diet and up the ante on your exercising, you may end up reducing blood glucose drastically, unless you verify the changing trend by estimating blood glucose and adjust the dosage of your anti-diabetics accordingly.

Long-standing diabetics, particularly those who also have high blood pressure and have not been able to achieve constant good control of blood glucose, are vulnerable to impairment in kidney function. If that happens, then their ability to eliminate anti-diabetic medications from the body gradually reduces. The pills accumulate in their body in high concentration, leading to a state of severe low glucose or hypoglycaemia. They can easily avoid such life-threatening situations by regularly monitoring their blood glucose as well as blood creatinine, an indicator of kidney function.

Diabetes is a progressive disease. With the passage of time, its severity inherently increases so one needs to gradually increase the dosage of one's anti-diabetic medications.

Please also remember that monitoring in the case of diabetes means much more than merely monitoring blood glucose. A diabetic needs to monitor several parameters such as weight, waist circumference, blood pressure, blood lipid levels, eye status, cardiovascular health and kidney function in addition to blood glucose monitoring. Let us discuss various tests used to monitor control. Some can be done by patients at home while others are carried out in pathology laboratories or doctors' clinics.

Home Test 1: Urine Glucose Estimation

Urine glucose estimation gives us a rough idea of blood glucose level while blood glucose estimation with glucose strips and a glucometer gives a more accurate estimate. In some situations, indirect estimation of blood glucose via urine glucose can be faulty. With glucometers now easily available, urine glucose estimation is rarely advised. However, even though it is almost obsolete, urine glucose estimation is still performed in some places, which is why this information is included here.

This is a simple test to be performed at home. If performed and interpreted correctly, it gives a rough idea of blood glucose level. However, it has many limitations and should not be solely relied upon to diagnose diabetes. On average, glucose is filtered from blood into urine when blood glucose level rises beyond 180 mg% so, usually in non-diabetics, there is no glucose in urine throughout twenty-four hours. The level of blood glucose beyond which it is filtered into the urine is known as 'renal threshold' for glucose. The interpretation of presence of glucose in urine is that, at that particular time, blood glucose is likely to be above 180 mg% provided the person's renal threshold is around 180 mg%.

The higher the amount of glucose in urine, the higher the blood glucose level is likely to be. Every person does not have a renal threshold of 180 mg% for glucose, though; a person with a lower renal threshold will have glucose in urine at blood glucose levels lower than 180 mg%, perhaps even at normal levels, while a person with a higher renal threshold will have glucose in urine only at blood glucose levels higher than 180 mg%. So, in patients with low/high renal threshold for glucose, rough indirect estimation of blood glucose can be faulty unless their renal threshold is known and factored in.

Precautions while doing urine tests at home

1. Use the dry strip method (Diastix) specific for glucose instead of Benedict's test, which gives false positive results, particularly in patients on Aspirin, Vitamin C, etc. To cut costs, split the test strip vertically to get two strips.
2. Completely empty the bladder fifteen minutes before the time of the urine test, so that when the second sample is collected for testing, you get freshly formed urine. This will give a more realistic idea of spot blood glucose value. In many diabetics, glucose is invariably spilled over in urine during the post-prandial period, yet they can have normal fasting blood glucose and absence of urine glucose in fasting state. However, in such patients, urine voided first thing in the morning is actually a mixture of urine formed over several hours overnight and hence can test positive for glucose even though urine actually formed in the morning does not contain glucose. So always collect freshly voided urine for glucose estimation.

3. Every time you do blood glucose estimation, test freshly voided urine so that you can also assess your renal threshold. As I said earlier, the normal threshold for glucose is 180 mg%, beyond which glucose enters the urine. However, many diabetics initially have a low renal threshold, which implies that glucose appears in their urine at blood glucose levels lower than 180 mg%. On the other hand, many long-standing diabetics have a high renal threshold for glucose. It is careless to increase or decrease medication dosage for such patients, based solely on urine glucose estimation.

Why do urine glucose testing at all, you might ask. Fair enough. Well, it is a tool for a diabetic to keep track of his day-to-day blood glucose values and get a rough idea about his own control. If there is a persistent change in the pattern of urine glucose levels, he should report this to his doctor.

Yes, blood glucose estimation is preferred over urine glucose estimation. However, an occasional patient is extremely averse to finger pricking by lancets. In such patients, urine testing is a pragmatic alterative method of self-monitoring. Something is definitely better than nothing.

MANY EXCEPTIONS TO THE RULE!

- Absence of glucose in the urine does not rule out diabetes. In many mild diabetics, fasting urine could be negative for glucose while post-prandial urine is more likely to be positive.

- On the other hand, the presence of glucose in the urine does not necessarily mean that the person is diabetic.
- Even if you have a reasonably good idea of your renal threshold for glucose, urine glucose estimation still cannot differentiate between normal blood glucose and low blood glucose (hypoglycaemia). Hence it cannot replace a blood glucose test.
- Do not rule out hypoglycaemia in a patient whose spot urine test is positive for glucose; he may not have voided urine for several hours.
- Absence of glucose in the urine does not mean the patient is 'well-controlled'—he could be 'over-controlled'.

Home Test 2: Self-Monitoring of Blood Glucose (SMBG)

A diabetic can self-monitor blood glucose by pricking a fingertip and getting a drop of blood on to the test area of a plastic test strip. The report is ready within seconds. You can get a rough reading directly in a range or with a specially designed palm-sized glucometer. The latter is, of course, more reliable and preferred over direct visual reading method based on colour change. With several brands of glucometers now available and affordable, visual direct reading of strips for very rough blood glucose value expressed in a range is almost phased out. However, if done properly, even this method is adequate to differentiate between hypoglycaemia and hyperglycaemia in emergencies or in case of sudden onset of new symptoms. Diabetics (particularly those who need repeated monitoring, such as pregnant diabetics), unstable diabetics, and those prone to hypoglycaemia should always keep a stock of strips handy, test blood glucose periodically, and keep a record for their doctor.

How reliable is self-monitoring of blood glucose?

SMBG is reasonably accurate and reliable, provided the strips are fresh and the meter is checked and recalibrated frequently. The strips should be stored in conditions recommended by the manufacturer. The person doing the test should be familiar with the procedure and the meter.

Precautions while doing blood tests at home

- Do not depend on SMBG solely for initial diagnosis, particularly if the readings are not unequivocally high and if the meter is not recently calibrated.
- Compare the results periodically with results from a standard method. While comparing, remember that spot method uses capillary blood so post-prandial values are higher by approximately 20 mg% as compared to those obtained with venous blood. Even in a fasting state, there can be a difference of up to 15 per cent between results

from a formal laboratory test done on venous blood and results from a home test done on capillary blood.

Glucometers are now available at around Rs 1000 per unit. This is affordable for many patients. I would recommend that every diabetic acquire a glucometer and use it for routine as well as SOS monitoring. The frequency of routine SMBG will depend on several factors including type of diabetes, degree of control and stability of control. Every patient should design his own plan in consultation with his doctor. For your ready reference, here is a baseline strategy:

1. All Type 1 diabetics, pregnant women with diabetes, severe type 2 diabetics who need more than 40 units of insulin per day and those with huge deviations in their blood glucose levels should undertake SMBG three times a day.
2. All well-controlled type 2 diabetics on 40 units of insulin or lower per day should undertake SMBG three times in the day but only on one or two days a week.
3. All diabetics on oral medications should undertake SMBG once a week or once a fortnight, each time three times that day.

Along with periodic testing, test blood glucose on SOS basis whenever there are sudden symptoms suggestive of hypoglycaemia as well as to verify glycaemic status during any acute emergency.

Out of the three times a day that you do SMBG, make sure that one is in a fasting state while the other two should be rotated to get a round-the-clock idea of blood glucose control. So, if you test your blood two hours after lunch and two hours after dinner one day, shift it around and test before lunch and before dinner the other day. In addition to this schedule, also test blood occasionally at 3 am, especially if you have typical hypoglycaemic symptoms or high fasting blood glucose despite taking over 20 units of long- or intermediate-acting insulin in the evening. Store the data generated from your SMBG regimen in a chart like the table shows and share it with your doctor on every follow-up visit.

Data from Self-monitoring of Blood Glucose (BG)

Date	Fasting BG	Pre-lunch BG	Post-lunch BG	Pre-dinner BG	Post-dinner BG	3 am BG	Random BG	Remarks	Insulin dosage
15/01/2013									
16/01/2013									
17/01/2013									

Note: All blood glucose values are in mg%; a similar format can be used for urine glucose test data.

HIGH FIVE

Five Ways to Master Your SMBG Technique

1. *Choose a good glucometer:* The latest glucometers have some distinct advantages over older ones: they yield results quicker, within five to seven seconds; they require much less blood; they do not require coding when you change over to strips made in different batches; and

their strip area with blood remains outside the meter so the meter does not get clogged. If your haven't already, do change over to a modern glucometer. Some leading brands are Bayer's Contour, Johnson & Johnson's OneTouch and Roche's Accu-Chek, and each has more than one model. Try to buy one that does not require coding, else there is the risk of you forgetting to recode whenever you start using a new vial made in a different batch. Purchase a glucometer locally but from an authorized source, so that you can enjoy servicing and a continuous supply of strips. Do not ask relatives to send or bring glucometers from overseas, as these may not be serviceable in India and their strips are often not available here. Also remember that strips of one brand are not compatible with others, and also that most brands have several models of meters and the strips of one model are not compatible with all other models of the same brand.

2. *Take care of the strips:* Store the strips properly, avoiding any contact with moisture by immediately closing the vial stopper tightly after taking out a strip. Do not use strips after the expiry date mentioned on the vial. There is an unopened expiry period of about six to twelve months, which means that all remaining unused strips should also be discarded at the end of that period. There is another expiry period for after breaking the seal, and this is usually shorter, about three months. This means

that once the seal is broken, you should use the strips within three months, after which all remaining unused strips must be discarded even if they are still within their unopened expiry period.

3. *Clean and dry your fingers well:* Wash your hands with soap and water and dry your fingers well before pricking. If your fingertips bear any remnants of any sweet that you ate before the test, the result will be enormously high. If your fingertips are not dry, the water will get mixed with the blood and the result will be enormously low. You can use alcohol (eau de Cologne, aftershave lotion or medicated alcohol) to clean your hands instead of soap and water. In that case, wait for a few seconds to allow the alcohol to evaporate, else you will end up testing diluted blood again.

4. *Get a proper blood drop:* Get an adequate-sized blood drop by using just adequate force with a lancet or no. 20 needles. If you prick the side of your finger and not the tip, you can reduce the discomfort because the sides are less sensitive than the tips. Do not squeeze with pressure, else some body fluids containing slightly lesser concentration of glucose may get mixed with the blood before it oozes out on to your fingertips. Always wipe out the first drop of blood, gently squeeze the finger again, and use the second drop of blood for the test—it is less likely to be contaminated.

5. *Cross-validate meter readings:* Do not trust a glucometer reading blindly. It is not a substitute for periodic laboratory testing. It should be used in between lab tests and during emergencies. Occasionally, but definitely, cross-check glucometer readings with laboratory readings; a difference of up to 15 per cent is acceptable. Also periodically cross-check with the control solution provided by the manufacturer along with the glucometer but do ensure that the control solution is not out of date.

Laboratory/Clinic-based Tests

Blood glucose estimation

Go in for laboratory-based fasting and post-prandial blood glucose testing every three months when you are stable. If you not stable, or if you have recently been diagnosed as a diabetic, go in for this testing more frequently. Here's a table to help you assess 'control':

Time	Blood glucose in mg% (plasma)		
	Good control	Fair control	Poor control
Fasting	<110	<140	>140
Two hours after meal	<140	<180	>180

Tests to detect kidney involvement

- Go in for an examination of urine for microalbuminuria in a pathology laboratory, which is more reliable than the dipstick method or 'micral' test. This test should be done only for those whose serum creatinine is normal and who do not have albumin in their urine when tested by routine method; estimating urine microalbumin in those who already have kidney impairment, which is confirmed by less sensitive tests, is a waste of money and time. This test should be done soon after type 2 diabetes is diagnosed and five years after type 1 diabetes is diagnosed. It should be repeated yearly till it is positive.
- Tests for serum creatinine, blood urea and blood urea nitrogen are blood tests to assess kidney function levels. Even though they are not sensitive enough to diagnose early kidney involvement, at least one should be done soon after diagnosis in type 2 diabetics and five years after diagnosis in type 1 diabetics (to get a baseline value). Subsequently, repeat the test at yearly intervals. Those with impaired kidney function should get tested more frequently.

Estimation of blood lipid levels (total cholesterol with high-density lipoproteins and low-density lipoproteins and triglycerides)

The first test should be done when you manage to control blood glucose after the initial diagnosis of diabetes. Thereafter, get these tests done at yearly intervals.

Detailed eye-check and electrocardiogram

You can get these done at yearly intervals, as long as they do not reveal any abnormalities. In people with diabetic retinopathy, eye examination should be done more frequently while in those with coronary artery disease or symptoms strongly suggestive of it also need specific investigations. In type 1 diabetics, the initial eye check-up should be done five years after diagnosis.

Routine physical examination

This should be done every three months in a clinic to track any changes in blood pressure, weight and waist measurement.

Special Blood Tests

Glycosylated haemoglobin (HbA1c) estimation (desired value <7%) is useful to estimate average control of blood glucose in the twelve weeks before it. As a good predictor of long-term metabolic control, it is also a good predictor of complications of diabetes. Blood can be drawn at any time of the day. If done by a reliable laboratory, it provides important information that blood glucose estimation cannot. Ideally, get it done every three months in addition to blood glucose estimation. The two values together give vital information. For example:

- *Normal HbA1c but high blood glucose:* The interpretation is that overall control over the previous twelve weeks has been all right but it is possible that control was lost a few days earlier or the patient did not take the previous evening's medication. It also raises the possibility of intermittent loss of control due to non-compliance. If the facts are verified, it would be prudent to increase medication dosage.

- *High HbA1c but normal fasting and post-lunch blood glucose:* The interpretation here is that overall control over the previous twelve weeks has been poor but control was achieved in the last few days.
- *Another possibility:* If a patient indulges in heavy evening snacking and / or heavy dinners but eats very lightly during the day in office (a common situation for those who live in the suburbs but work in downtown metro areas), the resultant high blood glucose values in the latter part of the day can be captured through SMBG. A combination of well-planned SMBG spanning all twenty-four hours and three- to six-monthly HbA1c testing is a very powerful tool in such cases to study blood glucose control and take corrective steps.

To avoid complications of diabetes, you must achieve 24/7 blood glucose control, and HbA1c is a good test to verify this. Normal fasting and post-prandial levels do not necessarily mean good round-the-clock control. If HbA1c is high despite good fasting and post-lunch values, it is likely that blood glucose values in the second half of the day are high. You can verify this via SMBG with glucometer. If confirmed, you must correct high pre- and post-dinner values via specific strategies like reducing afternoon/evening snacking or dinner, and adjusting the dosage of anti-diabetics taken around dinner.

Fructosamine test

Like HbA1c, this is a blood test. It gives information on average metabolic control over the previous two weeks. It is more useful than HbA1c to monitor diabetes during pregnancy. Only a few laboratories in India do it.

12

WHAT IS HYPOGLYCAEMIA?

Hypoglycaemia means low level of blood glucose (or blood sugar). In a normal person, fasting and post-prandial blood glucose values are in the range of 60–100 mg% and below 140 mg%, respectively. In the case of hypoglycaemia, blood glucose values plummet to below 50 mg%.

In diabetics who are untreated or inadequately treated, blood glucose values are higher than normal—that is a state of hyperglycaemia. However, if a diabetic who is dependent on insulin and/or medications to lower blood glucose does not take proper precautions, his blood glucose could fall into the hypoglycaemic range. In fact, of the various conditions in which a person develops hypoglycaemia, the most common is diabetes.

It is best to avoid hypoglycaemic reactions because, at times, they can be very dangerous, even fatal. Milder and repeated hypoglycaemia causes weight gain, which is harmful in the long term. To recognize hypoglycaemia early, and take prompt corrective action, you should gain a working knowledge of this condition.

You know that a diabetic has above-normal blood glucose, which is why he is given medications to bring it down into the normal range. When a diabetologist prescribes insulin or pills, he considers several parameters like the patient's age, physical activities, food intake and timing, weight and kidney function. Along with the medications, he also gives detailed dietary advice: what to eat, how much to eat, when to eat, how best to divide the total daily allowance of various food groups and so on. Diet and medication are carefully planned in such a way that the patient averts not only hypoglycaemia but also hyperglycaemia. You must meticulously follow the advice regarding dosage and timing of medication as well as timing, amount and type of food, and physical activity. There are no two ways about this.

WHAT IS HYPOGLYCAEMIA?

Hypoglycaemia means low level of blood glucose (or blood sugar). In a normal person, fasting and post-prandial blood glucose values are in the range of 60–100 mg% and below 140 mg%, respectively. In the case of hypoglycaemia, blood glucose values plummet to below 50 mg%.

Symptoms of Hypoglycaemia

The symptoms depend on the rate at which blood glucose is falling and the severity of the condition. As blood glucose starts falling below normal values, the bio-feedback apparatus detects this dip and automatically, hormones that counter the action of insulin are secreted into the bloodstream. The increased levels of these hormones in circulation produce symptoms such as palpitations, tremors, sweating and giddiness. These are the warning signals.

Then again, every diabetic will not develop all these symptoms during hypoglycaemia. He may get one or two of the ones mentioned here, but usually the same symptoms are repeated every time he has an episode of hypoglycaemia. These symptoms are known as adrenergic symptoms.

Even though mild hypoglycaemia is automatically corrected by the body, it is important to interpret adrenergic symptoms properly and take corrective measures to avoid severe hypoglycaemia. The reason is that if this natural measure is unable to elevate the blood glucose to normal levels, the brain will suffer from lack of glucose, for it is the only fuel that brain cells can utilize. If the brain is deprived of glucose, the patient will show symptoms of headache, confusion, abnormal behaviour and deteriorating level of consciousness, ultimately leading to coma. Some may have epileptic fits and the occasional patient may show symptoms resembling those of a paralytic stroke. These symptoms are known as neuroglycopenic symptoms.

Please remember that in some diabetics, particularly those that are elderly or have had the condition for a long time, the warning signals of adrenergic symptoms are absent. Such patients straightaway develop one or more neuroglyopenic symptoms and then usually need emergency hospitalization for treatment of hypoglycaemia.

How to Avoid Hypoglycaemic Reactions

No messing with meals

Always take food at fixed times. Never postpone food intake. Never reduce food intake. If, for some unforeseen reasons (such as non-availability of fuel for cooking), food is not ready at the specific time, take an equivalent quantity of ready-to-eat food, such as bread or biscuits.

Food in the backpack

When travelling, always carry some food in your personal baggage. This will help prevent hypoglycaemia in case food is not available at your scheduled time, due to unforeseen reasons such as a vehicle breakdown or flight delay.

Take the right dose

In case you are insulin-dependent and use vials and syringes, please be very careful about avoiding any mismatch between vials and syringes. (For details, please see Chapter 10.)

Prepare your body

Physical activity requires energy. Our body produces energy by burning glucose. If you are more active, you expend more energy, or more glucose. On days that you are likely to indulge in extra activity—say you have back-to-back meetings or a football match with colleagues—you should take an extra snack before you start the physical activity, to prevent the occurrence of hypoglycaemia.

Ban the booze

As far as possible, you should avoid alcoholic beverages. If you cannot avoid it, take alcohol in very small quantities and follow it up with food. You see, alcohol enhances the action of anti-diabetic medications so a diabetic who does not take his scheduled meal after taking alcohol is likely to have a hypoglycaemic episode.

Importance of Regular Monitoring

Even if your blood glucose is well controlled and steady, you should get it checked every three months and adjust the dose of insulin and/or pills as per the requirement, in consultation with your doctor. If blood glucose is well controlled, your doctor may reduce the dosage of your medications to prevent hypoglycaemia in the future.

You should also get your kidney function tested every year and more frequently if it is impaired. A commonly used test to evaluate kidney function is estimation of creatinine in blood. This test can be carried out along with a blood glucose test. If your kidney function is impaired, anti-diabetic pills are eliminated very slowly from the body. Their accumulation in the body can cause severe hypoglycaemia. Impaired kidney function is not uncommon in longstanding diabetics.

Remember that the pills are double-edged weapons and they should never be taken lightly. In fact, hypoglycaemia following some pills could be severe, prolonged, recurrent and tougher to treat than that resulting from inappropriate insulin administration. In case of significant impairment of kidney function, your doctor is likely to discontinue your pills and ask you to change over to insulin. Accept the change.

Self-monitoring of blood glucose or SMBG is an additional tool you can wield against hypoglycaemia. Regular monitoring will let you pick up the trend and give you an opportunity to adjust the dosage of anti-diabetic medications and/or food amount and timings while spot SOS monitoring will help you make an early diagnosis and take corrective action. (See Chapter 11 for details.)

Always carry an identity card on your person. This card should mention that you are a diabetic and that, if found ill, drowsy, or behaving abnormally, you should immediately be given sugar or fruit juice. The card should carry your name, address and emergency contact details.

How Best to Handle Hypoglycaemia

If and when you develop symptoms such as palpitations, sweating, tremors, and hunger—all suggestive of hypoglycaemia—you should immediately eat some ready snacks such as biscuits or a sandwich. If your symptoms are severe, immediately have 3 tsp of sugar or glucose. If you don't feel any better within fifteen minutes, have another 3 tsp of sugar or glucose.

If, however, you are being medicated with alpha glucosidase inhibitors (acarbose, miglitol, voglibose), then even a mild episode of hypoglycaemia should be treated specifically with glucose. In case you are on insulin injections, always keep a vial of glucagon injection handy. In case of severe hypoglycaemia, you or a family member can inject 1 ml of glucagon just like you inject insulin. It will help you recover immediately.

A dramatic recovery within a few minutes will confirm that you had hypoglycaemia. When you are better, analyse the situation to identify the possible underlying cause, such as missing or reducing food intake or not taking extra food before heavy physical activity or taking more than the prescribed dosage of medication. If you can spot the mistake, you can correct it. If the symptoms occur repeatedly, it is likely that your medication dosage needs to be reduced; you should consult your doctor. If the symptoms persist even after eating, it may not be hypoglycaemia at all, or it could be persistent hypoglycaemia. In that case, contact your doctor immediately.

Whenever your symptoms suggest hypoglycaemia, try to ascertain if you, in fact, have low blood glucose *before* reducing your medication dosage or eating extra food. Of course, if you are doubtful or if spot testing equipment is not available, you must take a light snack and reduce or avoid the next dose of your anti-diabetic medication and then contact your doctor to assess the situation and advise you.

Failure to recognize hypoglycaemia early and take corrective measures can lead to coma, particularly in elderly and long-standing diabetics. If it occurs at night, it is very hazardous for the caregivers may not discover it till the morning and prolonged hypoglycaemia can cause permanent brain damage.

All diabetics should take small, frequent meals and periodically monitor blood glucose levels even when everything is apparently fine. As they say, better safe than sorry!

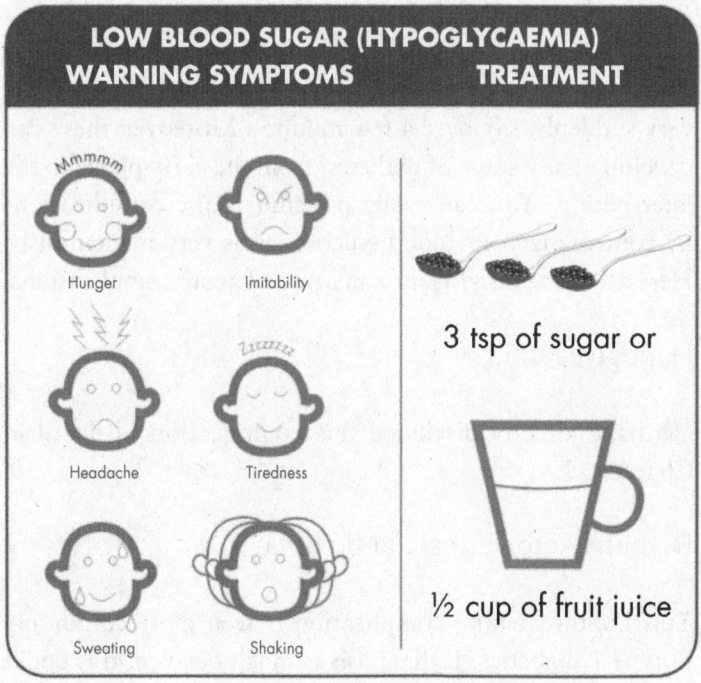

LOW BLOOD SUGAR (HYPOGLYCAEMIA)
WARNING SYMPTOMS   TREATMENT

Mmmmm
Hunger

Imitability

Headache

Zzzzzz
Tiredness

Sweating

Shaking

3 tsp of sugar or

½ cup of fruit juice

13

COMPLICATIONS OF
DIABETES

Diabetes is associated with several complications, some of them acute, which develop suddenly, and some chronic, which develop gradually over the long term.

Acute Complications of Diabetes

These complications, such as hypoglycaemia, can develop very suddenly, say over a few minutes. Moreover, these can develop at any stage of diabetes, from the early phase to the later period. You can easily pre-empt acute complications by controlling your blood glucose levels very meticulously. Here are some insights into an array of acute complications.

Hypoglycaemia

We have already discussed this complication in detail in Chapter 12.

Diabetic ketoacidosis and coma

This life-threatening complication is seen more commonly in type 1 diabetics. If diagnosis is much delayed, this could well be the first or presenting manifestation of diabetes in type 1 diabetics.

If diagnosis and treatment are not prompt, diabetic ketoacidosis invariably progresses to a coma or state of unconsciousness. It can develop in a known diabetic too, if treatment is withdrawn for a long time or if there is severe infection or a major stressful condition such as a heart attack.

Symptoms of ketoacidosis, like those of poorly controlled diabetes, are excessive thirst, excessive urination, severe exhaustion, sudden weight loss, deep and rapid breathing and slow deterioration in consciousness, ultimately leading to a coma as well as the symptoms of any other underlying disease such as tuberculosis (fever, cough, weight loss) or diabetic foot infection (severe pain, swelling, redness of affected area).

Some diabetics can develop ketoacidosis following a heart attack. In diabetics, chest pains or any discomfort characteristic of heart attacks are often absent so a sudden difficulty in breathing (symptomatic of ketoacidosis) could be the only manifestation of an underlying heart attack.

If a known diabetic experiences any dip in consciousness level over a period of a few hours, the family members or caregivers should suspect ketoacidosis and promptly seek medical help. While waiting for the doctor, you can perform random urine tests for glucose and ketones and/or a random blood glucose test. In such a situation, expect urine to be strongly positive for glucose and ketones, and blood glucose to be very high.

At times, hypoglycaemia may be mistaken for ketoacidosis. But remember that dip in consciousness is dramatic (within minutes) in the case of hypoglycaemia as opposed to gradual (over a few hours) in the case of ketoacidosis. Also, the coma state usually follows symptoms of poor control and the underlying condition (for instance, cough and fever in the case of tuberculosis or pneumonia) while hypoglycaemia can set in suddenly in an otherwise well-controlled patient. The above-mentioned home tests will help spot the difference. In hypoglycaemia, blood glucose is likely to be lower than 50 mg% and the urine is likely to be glucose-free. Being able to promptly differentiate between these two complications empowers caregivers in that they can treat hypoglycaemic episodes at home and avert hospitalization, which is a must in the case of ketoacidosis.

HOW YOU CAN AVOID DIABETIC KETOACIDOSIS AND COMA

Take your anti-diabetic medications regularly. Do not discontinue them, even on a sick day, unless your doctor specifically says so. Remember, even if a severe diabetic does not consume food, his blood glucose can rise as the liver produces more glucose in a state of severe insulin deficiency.

Undertake periodic self-monitoring of blood glucose at home with a glucometer and consult your doctor if two successive blood glucose values are high.

Monitor your blood glucose through laboratory tests every three months even when you are feeling perfectly all right and your self-monitored blood glucose values are steady. Do so more frequently during periods of inadequate control. Advance the test date if you are not feeling well. Stay alert for weight loss, frequent urination and excessive thirst.

If you are febrile or congested for more than a week, or if you develop a skin lesion that does not respond to basic medicines, inform your doctor. In fact, bring any new symptoms to your doctor's attention. This will help him diagnose the cause promptly and evaluate its effect, if any, on your diabetes.

Non-ketotic hyperosmolar coma

Unlike diabetic coma, which develops more commonly in type 1 diabetics, non-ketotic hyperosmolar coma (NKHOC) develops exclusively in type 2 diabetics, particularly elderly patients. It could also be the first manifestation of diabetes in an undiagnosed patient but it may also develop as a complication in a known diabetic. Some of the precipitating factors are heart attack, paralytic stroke, severe infection leading to septicaemia and certain medicines such as diuretics and mannitol. The affected person is severely dehydrated and

SYMPTOMS OF HIGH BLOOD SUGAR (HYPERGLYCAEMIA)

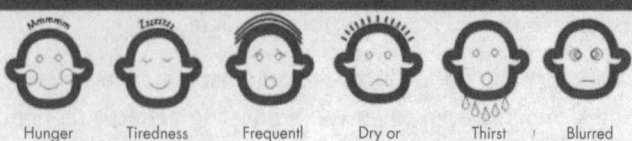

Hunger   Tiredness   Frequentl urination   Dry or itchy skin   Thirst   Blurred vision

Possible causes

- Not taking diabetes medication or taking too little, and/or taking at wrong time
- Eating too much or not eating the appropriate balance of food
- Illness or infection
- Trauma/stress: physical and/or emotional

What should you do?

- Test your blood sugar regularly
- Take your medication as prescribed
- Follow your meal plan
- Drink extra water
- Call your doctor if you continue to have high blood sugar

soon lapses into a coma, if he is not promptly diagnosed and treated. Blood glucose is extremely high (hyperglycaemia), usually between 600 mg% and 1000 mg%. NKHOC is a serious, life-threatening condition and demands immediate hospitalization.

Lactic acidosis

This is actually a complication of drug therapy and develops, very rarely, in diabetics being treated with oral pills of the biguanide class. It is extremely rare but supremely life-threatening. It often develops when a diabetic consumes biguanides despite their contraindication or consumes them in a dosage higher than normal. And then there are those even rarer cases—particularly in those on phenformin—when lactic acidosis can develop even in those that take them in proper dosage and for whom they are not contraindicated.

The symptoms are non-specific and usually include nausea, vomiting, and abdominal pain. Deep, rapid breathing develops subsequently and the patient may lapse into a coma. To prevent lactic acidosis, it is absolutely critical to strictly adhere to the correct dosage schedule and abide by any contraindication (please refer to Chapter 9.) If the caregiver is alert to the possibility of lactic acidosis, promptly withdraws the biguanides and admits the patient to a hospital equipped with good laboratories and intensive care and haemodialysis facilities, he can save the life of the affected diabetic.

Lactic acidosis is several times more likely to occur with phenformin therapy as compared with metformin therapy. Both are biguanides but there are subtle structural differences in their safety profiles. Phenformin has been withdrawn from most countries, including India, but metformin is the world's most popular and most widely prescribed anti-diabetic agent.

Chronic Complications of Diabetes

Among chronic complications, there are (1) specific complications comprising microvascular complications specific only to diabetes and (2) other complications including macrovascular disease and infections.

Microvascular complications

In patients with long-standing diabetes, particularly those with bad control of blood glucose, the capillary basement membrane (inner lining of microscopic blood vessels) is thickened and damaged. This leads to leakage of blood into the surrounding tissues. If the affected tissues are studied under the microscope, one sees a specific pattern of structural damage. This lesion is specific to diabetes and not reproduced in any other disease. The process mainly affects the kidneys (diabetic nephropathy), retina (diabetic retinopathy) and nerves (diabetic neuropathy). Diabetic microangiopathy is the umbrella term that covers all these conditions.

Metabolic and vascular abnormalities associated with poorly controlled diabetes cause the onset and progression of diabetic microangiopathy. This too can be prevented by early diagnosis of diabetes and tight control over blood glucose. It is important to achieve this goal because these complications undermine the quality of life gradually but seriously.

Diabetic nephropathy

This condition develops after about five years of persistently inadequate control of blood glucose. Once it sets in, kidney function gradually deteriorates (particularly if control is still poor) and ultimately the patient suffers from end-stage kidney failure. A major risk in this period is that of increased blood pressure. If blood pressure too is inadequately controlled, the deterioration of kidney function is accelerated. Once nephropathy sets in, high blood pressure poses a higher risk to the kidneys than high blood glucose. In fact, when kidney failure sets in, it is easy to control blood glucose. What you must concentrate on is strict control of blood pressure, initially to prevent nephropathy and subsequently to decelerate kidney function deterioration.

Diabetes is one of the commonest causes of end-stage kidney failure. In this stage, a diabetic is dependent either on repeated dialysis, usually three times a week, or a successful kidney transplant. Both alternatives are extremely expensive. It is vital to prevent diabetic nephropathy by controlling blood glucose and blood pressure religiously.

The most sensitive laboratory investigation to detect early involvement of kidneys is a urine test to detect microalbuminuria. Every diabetic should get this done on a yearly basis. Of course in those with significant kidney involvement, as indicated by rise in serum creatinine and blood urea nitrogen, there is no need to do urine testing for microalbuminuria. Today there are some very effective medicines of the angiotensin converting enzyme inhibitors and angiotensin receptor blockers families, which when given to patients with microalbuminuria lead to its reversal. All patients with microalbuminuria should be put on these agents to prevent further kidney damage.

Diabetic retinopathy

The retina, situated inside the eye, is the screen on which we register images of what we see. If it is damaged, sight is affected. Diabetes is a common cause of retinal damage leading to blindness.

Diabetic retinopathy develops in two stages, the first stage called pre-proliferative (or background retinopathy) and the second stage called proliferative retinopathy. Like diabetic nephropathy, it is very important to prevent retinopathy by controlling blood glucose strictly. If you are a diabetic, get your eyes thoroughly examined every year so that any changes can be detected at the earliest. In moderately advanced cases, further deterioration in eyesight can be prevented via laser photocoagulation treatment. This treatment is not curative but only helps prevent deterioration. If blood pressure is high, it must be controlled. Use of angiotensin converting enzyme (ACE) inhibitors,[1] even in normo-tensive diabetics, can also prevent diabetic retinopathy.

Diabetic neuropathy

Many long-term diabetics, especially those with poor control over a long term, suffer damage to their nerves. The symptoms depend on the functional type and anatomical site of the affected nerve. The nerves affected most commonly are those carrying sensations to the lower legs and feet, which is why lack of sensation in feet and legs is a common symptom. Because a person with diabetic neuropathy lacks

---

1 ACE inhibitors are used to treat high blood pressure, and can prevent deterioration in cases of diabetic retinopathy. Even if they are used in diabetics with normal blood pressure, the blood pressure will not fall significantly and yet good effects will be produced in the retina.

sensation in those areas, he is prone to repeated injuries to the soles and related secondary infections. It may even lead to gangrene, which usually leads to an amputation. Many patients complain of severe burning or tingling sensations. These symptoms are often severe enough to interfere with sleep at night, thus making the patient's life miserable. These people have a strange condition of 'painful but painless feet'. There are 'painful' symptoms but, at the same time, they lack pain and touch sensations.

Damage to autonomic nerves manifests in varied symptoms, depending on the nerves affected. Episodic vomiting and watery diarrhoea, particularly at night, are symptoms of autonomic neuropathy of the gut's nerve supply. Giddiness after a change of posture is common in elderly, long-term diabetics and indicates autonomic nerve disease of the circulatory system. A painless heart attack is another manifestation. Diabetics should get thoroughly evaluated if they develop difficulty in breathing or get tired even after minimal physical exercise: it could indicate heart failure. Many men with longstanding diabetes develop impotence, due to damage to the nerve supply of the penis.

Diabetic neuropathy can be prevented or considerably postponed if diabetes is diagnosed early and blood glucose is constantly controlled.

Once any microangiopathy sets in, the quality of life deteriorates significantly and the cost of medical treatment rises steeply. A diabetic must get totally involved in the management of his disease by acquiring information and updating it continuously. This will help him control blood glucose, prevent microvascular complications, and enjoy life despite diabetes.

Macrovascular diseases

These diseases affect the major arteries supplying oxygenated blood to various parts of the body. Atherosclerosis is a major macrovascular disease, and its prevalence is rapidly on the rise in India.

In atherosclerosis, the walls of major arteries are thickened and thus the internal diameter becomes narrow and irregular. This diminishes blood supply to the organ served by the affected artery/arteries and causes damage of the organ. To an extent, atherosclerosis is part of the ageing process but, in some people, it sets in prematurely and advances rapidly, leading to premature incapacitation, even death. Diabetes is a strong predisposing factor for the development and rapid advance of atherosclerosis. Depending on its anatomical site, macrovascular disease can affect various organs. More often than not, it affects multiple organs. Some important macrovascular diseases are described here.

Coronary artery disease (ischaemic heart disease)

Caused by the atherosclerotic narrowing of coronary arteries (which supply pure blood to the heart), this is the commonest type of heart disease. In some patients, symptoms start with anginal pain (discomfort or heaviness in the central part of the chest). Angina is aggravated by exertion and relieved by rest. At times, anginal pain starts even at rest, and this is the more dangerous variety. Some patients have heart attacks subsequently, particularly if they do not take care. In some patients, anginal symptoms are either absent or ignored; they seek medical attention only after a heart attack.

As mentioned, diabetes is an important predisposing factor for coronary artery disease. Diabetics are twice as likely to have heart attacks as non-diabetics. In post-menopausal diabetic women, the risk of a heart attack is four times higher than in post-menopausal non-diabetic women. Since diabetics are more likely to have painless heart attacks, implying that diagnosis is likely to be delayed, they are at higher risk. To prevent coronary artery disease, maintain ideal weight, waist circumference, blood pressure and blood lipid levels, and also avoid tobacco consumption.

Cerebrovascular disease

Caused by atherosclerotic damage to the blood vessels supplying blood to the brain, this disease manifests commonly as a paralytic stroke. Diabetics are two to four times more likely to suffer strokes than non-diabetics; moreover, they are likely to take longer to recover from a stroke. Hence, the emphasis should be on preventing strokes, using the same strategy as that to prevent coronary artery disease.

Peripheral vascular disease

Atherosclerotic affection of major blood vessels in the lower limbs leads to this disease. Affected people experience pain in the lower limbs, usually calves, when they walk. As the disease progresses, the pain sets in earlier and earlier and, in extremely severe states, there is pain even in a state of rest. If unchecked, peripheral vascular disease ultimately leads to gangrene, and the affected part needs to be amputated to save the patient's life. The site of amputation depends on the extent of atherosclerosis. In some cases, one toe is amputated while in more severe cases, an entire lower limb, above or below the knee, is amputated. Diabetes and prolonged tobacco consumption are two major underlying causes. Diabetics should strictly avoid tobacco in any form. Preventive measures are the same as those to be observed for other macrovascular diseases. Meticulous care should also be taken to safeguard the feet (see Appendix I).

A FOOTNOTE TO DIABETES

- As many as 25 per cent of diabetics develop a foot ulcer at least once in a lifetime. Some of these ulcers can develop gangrene, thus making amputation necessary.
- More than 50 per cent of non-traumatic lower limb amputations are done in diabetics.
- As many as 85 per cent of diabetes-related amputations can be prevented.
- Lower limb amputations are 15 times more common in diabetics than in non-diabetics.
- A significant 50 per cent of diabetics undergo at least one surgery in their lifetime, the most common ones being for foot infections and gangrene-caused amputations.
- Every 30 seconds, a surgery for diabetic foot disease is done somewhere in the world.
- About 20 per cent of hospital admissions in diabetics are for foot diseases.

High blood pressure (hypertension)

High blood pressure is extremely common in diabetics. In my experience, as many as 50 per cent of diabetics have high blood pressure compared with only about 15 per cent of the adults in the general population. Both diabetes as well as high blood pressure are independent risk factors of coronary artery disease, peripheral vascular disease and cerebrovascular disease. When diabetes and hypertension coexist, the risk is not merely added up but compounded.

When it comes to microvascular complications of diabetes, particularly nephropathy and retinopathy, hypertension intensifies these complications. In fact, in those with early nephropathy, hypertension carries more risk than high blood glucose, in the context of disease progression.

Blood pressure readings equal to or higher then 140 systolic and/or 90 diastolic indicate hypertension. A person must be totally relaxed, physically and mentally, during blood pressure measurements, else the reading may be elevated. Those with mildly elevated blood pressure should take the readings on two different occasions.

In diabetics, the two common types of hypertension are (1) essential hypertension and (2) renal hypertension. While there is no apparent underlying cause for the former, the latter is due to kidney involvement. Essential hypertension can precede or be diagnosed with or follow the diagnosis of diabetes. In fact, as per the current thinking, essential hypertension and type 2 diabetes are two faces of a common underlying disease. Renal hypertension in diabetes develops after the kidney is damaged by diabetic nephropathy; hence it always follows the onset of diabetes. In some patients, both types of hypertension coexist. Diabetics should bring their blood pressure down to 140/80 or less.

Infections in diabetics

Diabetics, especially those with poorly controlled blood glucose, have reduced capacity to fight infections. In fact, in an environment of uncontrolled diabetes, infections spread and rage like forest fires. Here are some common infections seen in diabetics:

Skin and soft tissue infections

Bacterial infections of the skin and the underlying fat, such as boils, cellulitis, carbuncles and abscesses, are common in diabetics. In fact, the symptoms of these infections, such as pain, swelling, and inflammation of the affected area, are often the presenting manifestations of diabetes. When diabetics with significant diabetic neuropathy and/or peripheral vascular disease develop bacterial infections in the feet or legs, these infections can spread rapidly and affect the deeper tissues, causing gangrene. This condition is called 'diabetic foot'. Fungal skin infections in sites such as the webbing between toes, one's groin, armpits and private parts are common in diabetics in the summer and monsoon. The skin gets darkened and scaly, and there is intense itching. Fungal infection of the oral cavity shows up as white patches in the buccal and palatal areas. These lesions are called 'oral thrush'.

Urinary tract infections

Infections of the urinary bladder and kidneys are common in diabetics. At times, these do not respond well to treatment and tend to turn chronic, in turn causing deterioration in kidney function.

Tuberculosis

Pulmonary tuberculosis (of the lungs) is common in uncontrolled diabetics, and tougher to treat than in non-diabetics. In fact, the coexistence of uncontrolled diabetes and tuberculosis is a grave situation.

Rhino-cerebral mucormycosis

This rare but life-threatening fungal infection enters the host's body through the nose, pierces the bony plate between the roof of the nose and the base of the brain, and spreads like wildfire inside the brain. Symptoms start with runny/blocked nose and progress into headaches, vomiting, high fever, convulsions and dips in consciousness. Classically seen in very poorly controlled and debilitated diabetics, it can lead to ketoacidosis.

14

DIABETES AND PERSONAL MATTERS

Can I Marry?

Of course you can! Like any other individual, a diabetic can marry and enjoy a happy married life. Of course, you should take your prospective spouse into confidence and inform him/her about your condition and all the possible complications that could arise as a result.

If it is possible, two people with established diabetes should not marry each other. This will ensure that at least one of the partners is in good health in their old age and thus able to care for the other. This will also relatively reduce the chances of their children developing diabetes.

There are extremely rare circumstances in which a diabetic should avoid marriage. If he has developed diabetes at a very early age (usually type 1 diabetes, rare in India) and exhibits severe complications like diabetic nephropathy or severe retinopathy leading to blindness, he should avoid getting married. This is because advanced complications diminish not only life expectancy but also compromise the quality of the remaining life, among other things by placing immense economic strain, and such a life may be rather unfair to his partner.

Will My Children Get Diabetes?

If one parent has type 2 diabetes, there is an approximately 25 per cent chance of the child developing the condition later in life. If both parents are diabetic, however, the likelihood rises to 75 per cent. Among children with one diabetic parent, those with a diabetic mother have slightly higher chances of developing diabetes. (Heredity plays a lesser role in type 1 diabetes.)

These are estimates for type 2 diabetes, however. Ultimately, whether a child develops diabetes or not depends on the interaction between environmental and hereditary factors. The former can be modified; the latter cannot.

Two children of the same parents can behave differently, depending on environmental factors. For instance, if one child is overweight, he is more susceptible to diabetes than his sibling who keeps obesity and diabetes at bay through regular physical exercise and prudent diet control. It is important to prevent diabetes in the next generation by helping your children avoid childhood obesity.

What Are the Risks If I Am Pregnant?

A woman with diabetes carries certain risk to herself as well as the developing foetus, particularly if blood glucose remains uncontrolled. Birth defects in various organs are more common in children of diabetic mothers. The correct way to significantly minimize the complications is to tightly control diabetes while using a temporary family planning measure and attempt to conceive after establishing blood glucose control. Diabetes in a man does not carry any direct risk to his wife during pregnancy, nor does it increase the chances of birth defects in the child.

Can I Satisfy My Partner Sexually?

Sexual drive in a diabetic woman is not significantly affected. However, longstanding diabetes in men, particularly if poorly controlled over the long term, can lead to organic impotence by affecting the nerves and blood vessels of the private organs. Many pills that reduce blood pressure can also cause impotence; high blood pressure is common in diabetics and they often require high doses of such pills.

A diabetic is also not immune to the psychological causes of impotence. As many as 35 per cent of diabetic men suffer from impotence, many of them silently because they are ashamed to talk about it even with their doctors. Impotence can interfere with a happy married life and the only way to avoid it is to keep blood glucose under persistently good control right from the day diabetes is diagnosed.

Impotence in diabetic men is treated by administering pills such as sildenafil (Viagra, for instance); implanting devices such as metallic implants or vacuum pumps to help overcome erectile dysfunction; and injecting drugs such as papaverine or alprostadil locally into the penis. A diabetic should frankly discuss any sexual impairment with his doctor and jointly plan appropriate treatment.

Can I Donate Blood?

Yes, you can. There is no blanket ban on blood donation by a diabetic. If your blood glucose is controlled and you are in good health, satisfying all the criteria that any prospective donor has to satisfy, you can donate blood. These criteria include absence of anaemia and uncontrolled high blood pressure. Both type 1 as well as type 2 diabetics can donate blood. In many western countries, those who have used insulin prepared from bovine sources are barred from blood donation to prevent the spread of animal-borne infections. However, over the last decade, the availability and use of bovine insulin have become nearly extinct there as well as in India.

Can I Travel?

In this supersonic age, the globe has really become a village and many people are on the move constantly. Many of these jetsetters are diabetic too. Long travel period, particularly to unknown areas and countries, can definitely cause problems for diabetics whose blood glucose is poorly controlled. A diabetic should postpone travel till he can establish good blood glucose control.

TRAVEL TIPS FOR DIABETICS

- Carry more than an adequate supply of medicines, keeping a buffer for unexpected delays in return. Your medicines may not be available in the places you are visiting or may require a prescription there. Remember, in developed countries, chemists do not issue medicines without a prescription from a doctor licensed to practise in that country. Moreover, in most foreign countries, the same medicines are several times more expensive.

- Carry a legible prescription along. In fact, request your doctor to write the genetic/chemical name of the medicine alongside the trade name. You may not be able to purchase your medicines overseas but the prescription will reveal your current treatment plan in case a doctor has to see you while you are travelling. If your case is complicated, it will be wise to carry a brief note from your doctor summarizing the current status of your health.

- If you are on insulin, request your doctor to also add a prescription for insulin syringes/pens and a note stating that you are required to self-monitor your blood glucose and must carry a glucometer and accessories (strips, lancets, cotton, spirit, etc.) in your personal baggage.

- You need not refrigerate insulin vials/cartridges in current use but do so for extra supplies. Never store insulin in the freezer compartment or take it to extremely cold places. If you do not have temperature-controlled storage facilities during your travel, wrap the insulin supplies in a few layers of thick woollen clothes (if the weather is extremely cold) or keep it in a dry earthen pot wrapped over with a wet towel (if the weather is extremely hot). If travelling by car, never keep insulin in the glove compartment or boot. When you leave the car for a pit stop, carry your insulin along, as a locked car can get very hot.

- Carry sufficient instant-energy foods (biscuits, chocolate, sandwiches, khakra, cream crackers) in your personal baggage. If you must travel for more than twenty-four hours, carry the equivalent of one full meal plus two snacks. For shorter visits, two snacks are sufficient. Your car may break down in the middle of nowhere. Your train may not arrive in time at a station where passenger meals are loaded. Your plane may not take off on time or in-flight food service may be disrupted by turbulence. If your meal is delayed for any reason, dip into your stock to prevent hypoglycaemia.

- Always wear comfortable shoes (leather or canvas). They should be broad enough to comfortably accommodate your toes. Never wear new shoes on a journey; break them in at least two weeks before your journey to avoid shoe bites. Always carry extra footwear and several pairs of seamless socks made of cotton or other absorbent material.

Can I Drive?

Of course, most diabetics can drive safely. Incidences of driving accidents related to diabetes are uncommon and not sufficient to justify a uniform ban on diabetics from driving. There are no blanket bans, though every country and regions within countries have framed rules and regulations that may differ to some extent. Diabetics regularly and safely drive their vehicles, even over long distances. However, you should be careful if you tend to have low blood glucose levels or visual impairment due to diabetic retinopathy, or if you have loss of sensation in your feet.

HOW CAN I PREVENT A DRIVING MISHAP?

- Diabetics, particularly those who are prone to hypoglycaemia should always carry their glucometer, accessories and appropriate snacks. The food supply should include items such as dextrose powder, chocolate, table sugar etc. for immediate recovery from low sugar state, as well as food items like biscuits and sandwiches for prevention of recurrence of hypoglycaemia.
- When embarking on long distance driving do random blood glucose estimation with a glucometer and take a snack such as biscuits or sandwiches if blood glucose is below 90 mg%.

- If and when you experience symptoms of low glucose, pull up the vehicle, measure your blood glucose level and consume dextrose, chocolate or table sugar if blood glucose value is below 70 mg%, or biscuits or sandwiches if blood glucose value is between 70-100 mg; wait till you are absolutely comfortable and then proceed.
- Have yearly eye check-ups to ensure that your vision is not impaired.

Can I Get a Job Easily?

Unfortunately, there is still rampant workplace discrimination against diabetics due to misconceptions in the minds of human resource professionals and medical officers of employers. Several organizations reject diabetics outright, without even considering that their medical condition will not impact on their job-worthiness at all. Diabetics should join forces to highlight this unfairness and take the help of experts in the field to sensitize workplace managements.

Diabetics whose blood glucose is usually reasonably controlled and who do not have advanced complications of diabetes can do most desk jobs and other light work. It has been reported in the UK that persons with diabetes take less sick leave than those who don't have it.

However, some professions are beyond the ambit of diabetics. In jobs where one needs to drive/fly/operate any

---

1 G.R. Kelman, 'Pre-employment medical examination', *Lancet* **11**: 1231–33.

vehicle, one must possess perfectly normal eyesight. A diabetic may not possess this and, a few years down the line, is more likely to suffer from impaired vision. Hence, diabetics are not considered for positions such as airplane pilots, train drivers or long-distance bus drivers. Also, working in lonely places or high altitudes is not suitable for diabetics.

Some of the outstanding people who shaped India's destiny were diabetics. Lokmanya Bal Gangadhar Tilak, Loknayak Jayaprakash Narayan and Ganesh Mavlankar, Speaker of the Constituent Assembly of India, are notable examples.

ECONOMIC COSTS OF DIABETES

Diabetes is associated with several chronic complications, treating which is much more expensive than treating diabetes. The costs of diabetes include:

- **Direct cost to patient and family** (medicines, supplies, laboratory tests, hospitalization, doctors' fees)
- **Direct cost to the health care sector,** particularly in the government and charitable sector (hospital services, laboratory services, health-care personnel)
- **Indirect cost to patient and family** (loss of working hours due to illness, handicaps, premature death, etc.)
- **Intangible cost to patient** (arising from anxiety, depression, pain, lack of self-esteem)

Diabetes is a very expensive disease. The WHO estimates that, between 2005 and 2014, India will lose 336.6 billion dollars from premature deaths due to heart diseases, strokes and diabetes. In the Indian context, where health insurance covers only 2 per cent of the population, most diabetics have to pay for treatment from their own pockets. The average annual cost of treatment of diabetes, as per work done at the M.V. Hospital for Diabetes and Diabetes Research Centre, Chennai, in 2010, was approximately Rs 26,000. Add to this the annual indirect cost of an average of Rs 5000. If one extrapolates these figures, India annually spends 31.9 billion dollars on diabetes care of its 62 million diabetics. (Contrast this with the US, which with 25.9 million diabetics, spends 174 billion dollars annually on direct and indirect costs.)

On an average, an Indian family with one diabetic member spends about 25 per cent of its annual income on managing the disease. Since India is a poor country (33 per cent of the world's poor live in India), this economic burden is unbearable for most Indian diabetics. Many have to raise funds by selling or mortgaging immovable assets and taking very-high-interest loans from the unorganized sector, since loans from banks and other financial channels are not available to them, for obvious reasons.

We must go all out to reduce this burden by preventing diabetes wherever and however possible and preventing complications of diabetes in those who already have it. This can be achieved by a combination of prudent lifestyle measures and appropriate medication. It is also vital to inform and educate the entire community about the punishing medical and economic implications of poorly controlled diabetes.

Should I Tell My Colleagues and Contacts about My Condition?

When you are being considered for a new job, ethics demand that the employer should ask personal questions (including your medical history) only after the decision to select you—subject to medical fitness—has been firmly taken.

There are no hard and fast rules about declaring your diabetic status. Take your decision after considering the pros and the cons.

Workplace woes

If you do not declare your diabetes, you will not be discriminated against at the time of initial recruitment, or later while being appraised for promotion. (This, of course, does not hold true in the case of certain positions, such as commercial pilots and armed forces personnel, for which diabetics are not considered at all. Pre-employment medical examination for these professions is very thorough and it is difficult as well as unethical to hide one's diabetes.)

If you do declare you have diabetes, however, you will be under scrutiny. In that case, if you have maintained good control over your blood glucose and if you do not have any complications, you will lead an absolutely normal life. When your colleagues see you leading a full life, they will gradually shed their prejudices against diabetics. Moreover, as they observe you and work with you, they will learn more about diabetes. You will thus sensitize the society to the challenges of diabetes.

Wedding blues

Young people of marriageable age, particularly young women and especially so in the case of arranged marriages, prefer not to disclose their diabetic condition so that they do not hamper their prospects of getting a suitable life partner. Do remember, however, that it is almost impossible to hide your diabetes from your spouse over the long term. You will need medication, you will need insulin injections, you will need frequent medical check-ups—how do you propose to explain all those away? Do consider the implications of your decision.

The good news

Whether it is before a job interview or a wedding ceremony or generally, if you do declare to one and all that you are indeed a diabetic, you will be free forever from the tension and anxiety associated with hiding your condition from others. It cannot be too much fun to rush to the toilet to take your medication or to eat at odd times to prevent or treat hypoglycaemia or hide vein puncture marks while struggling to explain ('Oh, I went for a routine check-up') or always avoiding desserts at official or social meals ('Oh, I'm on a diet').

Am I Eligible for Life and Health Insurance?

Life and health insurance are absolutely essential for everyone, including diabetics. However, both are grossly undervalued in India. It is not surprising that only 20 per cent of insurable Indians actually have life insurance. The status of health insurance is even more dismal; only 2 per cent of Indians have health insurance. We do not have figures for health insurance cover in the diabetic population but we can safely assume that these are obviously worse, for these policies are not easily available to diabetics.

Life insurance

Don't worry. There is no blanket exclusion for diabetics from all life insurance policies. Let us accept, however, that diabetics will have to pay stiffer premiums as compared with non-diabetics. Also, there are some limitations (features, duration) to the type of policies available.

If you are diabetic or if your diabetes is detected during the pre-policy medical examination, the life insurance company will ask you to undergo in-depth assessment of your blood glucose control and tests to diagnose complications such as kidney, heart and eye diseases. If you have significant complications, it is needless to say that you will not get a life insurance policy. However, since life insurance is essential, diabetics should shop for and get the best possible policy.

In general, it is rather difficult for type 1 diabetics (2 per cent of diabetics in India) to get life insurance policies. Type 2 diabetics have a bunch of options. Here are some tips to help you make the most of what life insurance companies offer:

1. Buy life insurance at a young age when you are less likely to suffer from diabetes and other chronic diseases. At a young age, you also get the advantages of wider choices and lower premiums.

2. Always pay your premium on time to keep the policy live. If you apply for renewal after defaulting, you will have to undergo a medical examination and there is a risk that you may have developed diabetes or other chronic complications in the interim.

3. If you have diabetes, better late than never: buy life insurance policy as early as possible when the complications of diabetes are unlikely to have developed. Study the plans offered by different companies and opt for the best bargain. Policies offered to diabetics are generally of a shorter duration. Keep your blood glucose levels and HbA1c under tight control to minimize/avert complications. This will help you to get discounts in your yearly premiums and also help you buy new policies.

Health insurance

Did you know that there are customized health insurance policies for diabetics? Usually available for five-year terms, these are offered after thorough medical and pathological tests to rule out any existing complications. If you have significant complications or poor blood glucose control, insurance companies are very likely to reject your application.

If you develop diabetes-related complications like kidney/ heart/eye disease or need foot/leg amputation during the operational period of the policy, the insurance company makes a down payment as per the terms. Do remember though that every policy stipulates a time period at the beginning of the policy during which you are not covered for such complications. Since these are short-term policies, you will have to buy a new policy at the expiry of the existing policy. The new policy will be issued only after the insurance company makes sure that you do not have any complications.

Type 1 diabetics do not get health insurance policies in most countries, including India, if they apply individually. However, they have a chance to buy group insurance through their employers.

> Never conceal your diabetic condition when purchasing a new life or health insurance policy.

A word of caution

Many people, especially in India, tend to hide their condition of diabetes and high blood pressure from insurance companies. Now, even if one is smart and meticulous, it is difficult to hide these conditions during critical illness. You cannot avoid mentioning your condition to your doctors, can you? Even if you have not disclosed your condition to the insurer, you are wise enough to know that hiding medical information from doctors, particularly during severe illness, is detrimental to your health. And so, these conditions and complications are recorded in hospital documents when a patient gets admitted for emergency treatment. At times, if the person is too ill to narrate his medical history, doctors get the history from close relatives.

Now, consider this. A life-insured person succumbs to his illness and relatives claim the insured amount. The insurance company obtains a copy of his entire hospital records and tallies the medical history with the one available in their records. If there is the slightest discrepancy, the insurance company absolves itself from paying the assured amount, quoting agreed terms and conditions of the policy. When the hospital records highlight diabetes and the company records draw a big blank on that front, you can only imagine the discrepancy and the consequences.

When a health-insured person gets hospitalized, narrates his true medical history, recuperates, gets discharged and then files an application with his health insurance company for reimbursement of hospital expenses, what happens? The company obtains his medical records from the hospital and tallies the recorded history with its own records. Enter discrepancy, exit reimbursement!

Let me share two real-life stories to explain these ideas better.

Case 1: Never withhold information to escape premiums

When he was thirty-nine, Pratap signed on for a long-term policy with a well-known life insurance company. He had been diabetic since the age of thirty-five but he concealed this fact to save on extra annual premium charges, which he would have to pay due to his diabetes. Unfortunately, at forty-three, Pratap died following a massive heart attack. Since the policy was active when he passed away, his wife claimed the insured amount. Pratap's hospital records revealed that Pratap had been suffering from diabetes for four years when he purchased the policy. Since diabetes can indirectly make a patient vulnerable to ischaemic heart disease, the insurance company rejected the claim on the grounds that the patient had not shared vital medical information. As a result, even though Pratap's life insurance policy was active at the time of his death, his family had to face financial hardship.

Case 2: Always read the fine print

Ganesh is sixty-seven. He has had diabetes for twenty years. At the age of fifty, he signed on for health insurance policy on the advice of a smooth-talking agent who mentioned all the benefits of the policy but conveniently left out the fact that Ganesh should share details of his existing diseases with the insurance company. Ganesh's mistake was that he did not read the application form carefully. He missed out on several terms and conditions in fine print, blindly signed on the dotted line, issued the cheque and relaxed. Needless to say, he did not declare his diabetes in the application form. For seventeen years, Ganesh religiously renewed his policy by issuing timely annual cheques to the insurance company. Now, over this period, Ganesh acquired complications of diabetes such as ischaemic heart disease, high blood pressure and urinary tract infection. Six months ago, Ganesh had to be hospitalized in severe distress, as he could not pass urine. Doctors advised him to go in for prostate surgery to relieve his urinary obstruction. After controlling his various complications and stabilizing him, doctors performed prostate surgery. Ganesh finally went home after two weeks.

Due to diabetic complications, Ganesh had to spend nine extra days in the hospital, incurring heavy expenses. He had a tough time generating the cash to settle the hospital bills. He thanked god for giving him the foresight to buy a health insurance policy. Soon after being discharged, Ganesh filed for reimbursement. One fine day, he received a letter from the insurance company. He expected a cheque but was shocked to find a claim rejection instead! The insurance company informed him that his claim had been rejected because he had withheld information about his diabetes at the time of buying the policy. The insurance company had discovered Ganesh's diabetic condition from the records pertaining to his hospitalization.

In due course, Ganesh recovered from the shock, accepted his blunder, cursed the insurance agent and launched damage control. He pleaded with the insurance company for part reimbursement, arguing that an enlarged prostate is not a complication of diabetes and requesting reimbursement for expenses relating to five days of hospitalization (conceding that the nine extra days were required due to his diabetes and associated complications) and surgery-related fees. The insurance company rejected his plea again.

Should I Stop My Diabetes Medication When I Fall Ill Otherwise?

As if the complications of diabetes are not enough, you are pretty likely to fall sick with any of the host of viral and bacterial diseases on the rampage all around us. On days of such other illnesses, you must not discontinue your regular anti-diabetic medication without consulting your doctor.

A person with uncontrolled diabetes produces a large amount of glucose in his liver. Hence, even if he does not eat or drink, he is likely to have high blood glucose during the illness. Moreover, the stress of underlying illness tends to elevate blood glucose. In a severe and uncontrolled diabetic state, you may experience symptoms of nausea, vomiting, abdominal pain and reduced appetite. Under such circumstances, you may tend to stop medication. This may lead to further rise of blood glucose and may even precipitate a diabetic coma.

To avoid misinterpreting your blood glucose status, you should repeatedly monitor your urine for ketones and blood glucose at home on sick days. If you have any doubts, do not hesitate to contact your doctor and verify your blood glucose level by the conventional lab method. These instructions are particularly critical for severe diabetics who need insulin or strong oral medication.

IDENTITY/INFORMATION CARD

All diabetics, especially those who are elderly and those prone to episodes of low blood sugar, must always carry an identity/information card on their persons. It is also smart to staple a small sachet of glucose or powdered sugar along with the card. Should you need an instant energy fix or experience a hypoglycaemic state while you are at work or on the road or away from your medication, this could be a lifesaver.

Front

DIABETIC PATIENT IDENTITY CARD

My Name: ....

Blood Group: ....

Address: ....

....

Phone Res.: .... Off.: ....

My Doctor's Name: ....

Clinic address: .... Phone Res.: ....

Clinic: ....

I am on the following medicines: ....

....

Back

AN
APPEAL FOR HELP

I am diabetic. If I am found ill or fainting or
behaving abnormally please give me some sugar
(about two tablespoonfuls) in water or a sweet drink.
If this does not revive me,
please take me to a hospital or a doctor.
Your care may save my life

15

MYTHS AND TRUTHS ABOUT DIABETES

As you know by now, in my model of diabetes management, knowledge plays a vital role. In fact, it plays a pivotal role. Knowledge is the catalyst that motivates a diabetic to take control of his lifestyle and his disease and sensitizes a non-diabetic to the many manifestations of the disease in the patient, in interpersonal relationships and in social interaction. A very important part of knowledge is busting myths to get to the truth. Many people have many misconceptions about diabetes, and that is detrimental to the goal of managing the condition. Here are some myths and truths about diabetes . . .

Myths about the Prevalence of Diabetes

Myth 1: Diabetes is a disease of the rich, and mainly found in western countries

Truth
Diabetes is prevalent all over the world. It has no geographic, religious, socio-economic or any other limitations. Obesity, which is more common in financially better-off people, is a predisposing factor for type 2 diabetes and so the condition is more evident in obese people. However, in India, a large number of diabetics have average or below-average

weight. And, in many of the underprivileged and seriously underweight citizens, diabetes remains undetected for way too long due to lack of medical facilities or lack of access to them.

Myth 2: India is the diabetes capital of the world

Truth
India is not the diabetes capital of world—China is. India has the world's second largest population of diabetics. As per 1995 estimates by the International Diabetes Federation, India had apparently surpassed China and gained the dubious distinction of being the world's diabetes capital. In 2010, however, through a comprehensive and systematic survey employing super-sensitive diagnostic criteria, the Chinese found that they had 91 million diabetics, a figure much higher than that projected by earlier surveys and also much higher than the number of diabetics in India. In 2011, the Indian Council of Medical Research undertook a survey and declared that India had 62.4 million diabetics. This figure was much higher than the earlier projected figure, yet much lower than the Chinese figure. Currently, China is the world's diabetes capital.

Myth 3: If you shun sweets, you won't develop diabetes

Truth
Diabetes develops as a result of the interplay between hereditary and environmental factors. Diabetics have a

deficiency of insulin, the hormone responsible for controlling blood glucose. Insulin is produced in the pancreas. Anyone who develops moderate to severe insulin deficiency will have diabetes even if he does not eat any sweets. And yet, this does not mean that a diabetic can eat as many sweets as he wants. A diabetic should shun all foods containing sugar, and opt for foods containing artificial sweeteners such as sucralose and aspartame.

Myth 4: You cannot get diabetes if no family member has it

Truth
To reiterate, diabetes is a result of both hereditary and environmental factors. It may not necessarily express itself in every generation. Moreover, who knows you may have, or had, a relative whose condition stayed undetected all his life. It can happen in mild diabetics.

Myths about the Diagnosis of Diabetes

Myth 5: A urine sugar test is enough to rule out diabetes

Truth
Absence of sugar in the urine does not always rule out diabetes because mild diabetics do not pass sugar in their urine throughout the day and fasting urine may thus be devoid of sugar. Urine passed two hours after a full meal or a 75 gm

glucose load is more likely to have sugar as compared with urine passed in the morning.

Myth 6: Sugar in the urine confirms diabetes

Truth

In some conditions, like those listed below, sugar is present in the urine even if the patient is not a diabetic. These conditions should be ruled out before diagnosing diabetes:

1. In pregnant women, urine contains lactose, which tests positive for urine sugar in Benedict's test.[1]
2. In people taking drugs such as vitamin C, para-aminosalicylic acid and aspirin, false positive results are likely with Benedict's test for urine sugar.
3. In people with a low renal threshold, glucose is present in the urine even when the blood glucose level is in the normal range.

It is always advisable to test blood glucose, and not urine glucose, to confirm the diagnosis of diabetes. Fasting blood glucose below 100 mg% and post-glucose-load blood glucose below 140 mg% rules out diabetes, whereas values above 126 mg% and 200 mg% (respectively) confirm it. If post-glucose values are between 140 mg% and 200 mg%, the condition

---

1 Though completely outdated, Benedict's test is still used occasionally as it is inexpensive. While modern strip tests specifically detect the presence of glucose in the urine (present in uncontrolled diabetes), this test detects the presence of reducing substances. Hence, sugars other than glucose as well as certain drugs test positive.

is impaired glucose tolerance. These people are not diabetics but require frequent check-ups, as many do develop diabetes in a few years.

Myth 7: Only a complete glucose tolerance test can verify blood glucose control in a diabetic

Truth

Complete glucose tolerance test (GTT) is not only cumbersome but also rather costly and not at all necessary to monitor blood glucose control in a known diabetic. Fasting and post-prandial blood glucose values are sufficient. Moreover, in most patients, GTT is not required for the initial diagnosis of diabetes.

Myth 8: If there's no sugar in the urine, diabetes is well controlled

Truth

Mild diabetics may not pass sugar in their urine throughout the day; usually sugar appears in the urine when blood glucose is above 180 mg%. Moreover, many long-standing diabetics have a high renal threshold: this means that they do not pass sugar in the urine even though their blood glucose is higher than 180 mg%. Occasionally, we come across a patient whose urine is devoid of sugar even when blood glucose is as high as 225–250 mg%.

In fact, urine examination is inadequate from another perspective too. With a few exceptions, the inference of absence of sugar in urine is that the blood glucose at that particular time is below 180 mg%. However, a urine examination does not tell us the exact blood glucose value. It could be anywhere from 175 mg% to 40 mg%. A urine examination alone is not sufficient to differentiate between good control, over control and inadequate control of blood glucose level. You must undergo periodic blood glucose examination—every three months in well-controlled diabetics and more frequently in initial stages and in poorly controlled diabetics.

Myth 9: Diabetes can be cured

Truth

Unfortunately not. Unlike diseases caused by viruses and bacteria, diabetes has no cure. You can only keep diabetes in check by keeping your blood glucose levels under control.

Once in a while, we come across a patient who says, 'I had diabetes some years ago but I was cured last year and have not followed it up with the doctor.' These are most likely cases of stress-related diabetes. Some people develop diabetes during periods of extreme stress such as a major surgery, accident or infection. Their blood glucose values normalize when the stress is over. These people may claim that they have been 'cured' of diabetes. However, they are quite likely to develop diabetes in future, whether they are subjected to stress or not. They should get their blood glucose tested regularly and religiously even if they show no classic symptoms of diabetes.

Myth 10: You should stop your medication on the day of your blood glucose test

Truth

In all diabetics except those with very high blood glucose and type 1 diabetics, doctors always begin treatment with dietary restrictions and physical exercise. They do not start you off on insulin or anti-diabetic pills immediately. Drugs are added to the regimen later for patients who do not respond to less-invasive measures. This implies that, in these patients, blood glucose will rise immediately after they stop insulin or pills and they will not be able to control their blood glucose 'naturally'. It is for this reason they should never stop medication on the day of blood glucose estimation, for that would defeat the very purpose of assessing whether the treatment is adequate and whether the dosage needs to be increased or reduced. In case you did not take your morning medications/insulin on the test day, do tell the doctor while you show him your blood glucose report.

Myth 11: Diabetics on insulin and medication do not need strict diet control

Truth

This is a fairly common misconception and it is responsible for poor blood glucose control in many diabetics. Dietary discipline is the very mainstay of diabetes management. Never ever take it lightly.

Myth 12: Diabetics should not eat rice

Truth

This concept is outdated and plain wrong. Chemically, there is not much difference between the composition of rice or wheat or other cereals for that matter. They contain complex carbohydrates, which are gradually digested and slowly converted into glucose. One can always exchange (substitute) a wheat preparation for one prepared with an equal amount of rice or another common cereal, as long as the cereal consumption does not exceed the daily allowance. Also, just like cereals, leafy greens and fresh fruits are very beneficial for diabetics as they provide considerable roughage.

Myth 13: It is all right for diabetics to drink alcohol

Truth

As far as possible, diabetics should avoid drinking alcohol regularly. An occasional drink does not do any harm, provided that you

- avoid accompanying high-calorie foods such as nuts, wafers, fried poppadums, cheesy nachos, etc.
- calculate the amount of calories you consume in drink and reduce it from other foods. (As an example, 250 ml of beer or 30 ml of whisky yield 110–120 calories, which is the equivalent of three slices of bread. So you know what not to eat later!)

Diabetics should note that alcohol enhances the blood glucose lowering action of oral pills and may reduce blood glucose to a dangerously low level, particularly if you skip a meal after a few drinks. Lactic acidosis, a rare but dreaded side effect of phenformin and metformin (blood glucose lowering pills of the biguanide class), is more likely to occur in those who consume alcohol. Some diabetics being treated with chlorpropamide (blood glucose lowering pill of the sulphonylurea class) develop severe facial flushing every time they consume alcohol.

Myth 14: Rock salt is okay whereas regular salt is not

Truth
Chemically, there is no difference between regular salt and rock salt. So, if you have been asked to restrict your salt intake, it goes for rock salt as well. Many diabetics with associated high blood pressure and heart problems are advised to go easy on the salt.

Myth 15: Diabetics can binge on polyunsaturated fats

Truth
Yes, polyunsaturated fats (safflower oil, sunflower oil, soybean oil, corn oil, cottonseed oil) and saturated fats (animal fats) yield equal calories. Yes, consuming the former does not elevate blood cholesterol significantly. But no, this

does not mean that you can consume polyunsaturated fats limitlessly. After all, they are concentrated sources of energy and cause weight gain and loss of blood glucose control, if you exceed your daily quota. Moreover, some oils rich in polyunsaturated fats have an unfavourable w6:w3 fatty acid ratio (please refer to Chapter 7).

Myth 16: Ayurvedic medicines are very effective and safe

Truth

Many people use Ayurvedic medicines and supplements to manage diabetes. Claims about their efficacy and safety have not been ratified by well-designed clinical trials. Jamun powder, methi seeds and karela juice are some home remedies, while there are many expensive branded products as well. Jamun (jambul fruit), methi (fenugreek) and karela (bitter gourd) have very mild blood-glucose-reducing properties, which by itself is inadequate except in very mild diabetics for whom diet control and physical exercise will work just as well.

Often, these medicines are prescribed along with standard allopathic ones. While allopathic medicines actually reduce blood glucose, Ayurvedic medicines get the credit. However, these medicines cannot replace insulin or allopathic oral pills in the management of diabetes. I know several patients who have changed over to these medicines and returned to me in a worse state, only to regain control on shifting back to insulin or allopathic anti-diabetic tablets.

Myths about Insulin

Myth 17: Once you're on insulin, you're always on insulin

Truth

Not at all. Some type 2 diabetics may need insulin only during acute infections or complications and can revert to their earlier insulin-less therapy once the acute illness is over.

Myth 18: Insulin frequency is increased if diabetes worsens

Truth

Not always. By splitting the insulin dose, you can get better control of diabetes and also avoid hypoglycaemia. This may be the reason why the doctor suggests that you take two daily insulin injections rather than one.

Myth 19: Type 2 diabetics never need insulin

Truth

During illness and stress periods, or if the oral drugs become ineffective, type 2 diabetics will need insulin.

Myth 20: If you take insulin regularly at the same time in the same dosage, you cannot get an insulin reaction

Truth

Insulin reaction (hypoglycaemia) can also occur due to variations in diet, exercise, metabolic control of diabetes, site of injection and type of insulin. You must go in for frequent blood sugar tests to ensure that you do not develop a tendency for hypoglycaemia.

Myth 21: Insulin bottles must be stored in a refrigerator

Truth

Not at all. You can safely store an insulin bottle in use at room temperature but take care to keep it away from direct sunlight and heat-producing gadgets. Even in summer months in extremely hot areas, insulin bottles can be safely stored in earthen pots covered with a wet cloth.

16

CAN I PREVENT DIABETES?

Prevention is so much better than treatment, more so for a disease like diabetes, which has multifaceted complications that can seriously undermine lifespan and life quality. Unfortunately, it is not possible to prevent every subtype of diabetes in every potential diabetic. However, if we are pragmatic and far-sighted both as individuals and as a community, we can considerably reduce the prevalence of type 2 diabetes. In some cases, even though we cannot prevent it, we can postpone the onset and reduce the severity. Here are some suggestions and ideas to plan your strategy to prevent diabetes:

Pre-empt to Prevent

As soon as you turn thirty, you should make it a point to monitor your blood glucose levels periodically. Unless you experience any complications, you can schedule this test once every two years. Increase the frequency to yearly if the baseline values are on the higher side of normal and to half-yearly if the values fall in the impaired glucose tolerance (IGT) range.

Watch for the Signs

If you have a family history of diabetes in first-degree relatives or if you are overweight/obese or if you suffer from premature onset of high blood pressure and coronary artery disease, you should not wait till you turn thirty. Schedule your glucose-monitoring blood tests at the age of twenty.

Undo the Damage

Many people with diabetes pass through the IGT stage—also known as pre-diabetes—before they become established diabetics. How long you classify as a pre-diabetic is dependent on several factors and the period varies with individuals. It is in this neither-here-nor-there state that you have your best chance of reverting your blood glucose levels to normal and safe range, all through prudent lifestyle measures. It is vital to undo the damage as soon as possible to pre-empt any risk of macrovascular diseases, which set in at the IGT stage.

Watch Your Weight

Needless to say, if you can avoid becoming obese, you can avoid getting diabetes. Healthy living includes regular physical exercise, prudent planning of meals, and avoidance of stress. Your body's own insulin works much better when you are in the normal weight range than when you are overweight. In other words, by maintaining your weight in the normal range, you can extract extra mileage from your own insulin and thus reduce the chances of your developing diabetes.

Nourish the Child

It has been amply proved that if a child faces protein malnutrition in the uterus as well as in infancy and childhood, it damages the beta cells in his pancreas, leading to insulin deficiency and diabetes in the future. Such malnutrition-caused diabetes can be prevented by improving nutritional status not only during infancy and childhood but also during intra-uterine growth. To a great extent, this is more of a socio-economic issue and hopefully the situation will improve in the near future.

CAN I POP A PILL TO PREVENT DIABETES?

As of now, there is no magic bullet to prevent diabetes, though research is under way to establish whether various medicines currently used in the impaired glucose tolerance (IGT) stage can help prevent or postpone the onset of diabetes. Some of these pills, such as metformin and acarbose, have been used with moderate success (along with other measures described in this chapter) to stop impaired glucose tolerance (IGT) from turning into diabetes.

In a major research project completed in September 2006, the drug rosiglitazone proved to be extremely effective in preventing type 2 diabetes in people diagnosed with IGT.[1] When compared with earlier studies, the results were twice as good as those obtained with acarbose and metformin. Titled 'Dream', the study included 5269 pre-diabetics, half of whom were treated with 8 mg of rosiglitazone daily for three years while the other half were treated with 15 mg of ramipril, a drug with the potential to prevent diabetes. The use of rosiglitazone resulted in a 62 per cent risk reduction for the development of diabetes as compared with a 9 per cent risk reduction in those on ramipril. However, rosiglitazone has been withdrawn from markets in most countries following the observation of higher chances of heart attacks and sudden death in patients on rosiglitazone as compared with other anti-diabetics. (For details, see Chapter 9.)

Recently, pioglitazone, a drug with properties similar to rosiglitazone, has been shown to be effective in preventing the onset of diabetes in pre-diabetics. In a project titled 'ACT NOW', 602 patients participated for 4.2 years. Half received pioglitazone and half received a placebo. Those on pioglitazone had 72 per cent less chance of developing diabetes during the period compared with those on

---

1 For details, see the publication of the study and its results in *Lancet* **368**, pp. 1096–1105.

placebo.[2] However, it is under surveillance as it is suspected to cause cancer of the urinary bladder.

While newer drugs are being researched and declared fit for consumption, pre-diabetics who do not follow or respond to diet and exercise regimentation can opt for metformin or acarbose to prevent diabetes. The role of metformin in preventing diabetes has been evaluated in a study done in India by Ramachandran. Done over thirty months, the study covered 531 pre-diabetics. Patients on metformin had 26.7 per cent lesser chances of developing diabetes during the study period compared with those on placebo.

Type 1 Diabetes: Prevention and Remission

Considerable progress has been made in preventing type 1 diabetes. It is now possible to identify potential type 1 diabetics by looking for specific markers of the disease. Siblings of patients who have been recently diagnosed as type 1 diabetics have increased chances of having auto-antibodies, which a blood test can detect. It is known that those who have these antibodies develop type 1 diabetes within a period of a few months to three years. To prevent this, siblings of recently diagnosed type 1 diabetics should be screened for

2 R.A. DeFronzo, 'Pioglitazone for diabetes prevention in impaired glucose tolerance', *New England Journal of Medicine* **364**(12): 1104–15.

these antibodies and those who test positive should be treated for prevention of diabetes. Drugs like nicotinamide, certain vaccines and very low dose insulin injections have shown promise in this context.

As for inducing remission (a state of reversal of the disease) in those already diagnosed as type 1 diabetics, there has been very encouraging progress. If immunosuppressive pills are administered as early as possible—within four weeks after diagnosis of type 1 diabetes—many patients can achieve remission. In some, blood glucose levels can be normalized without insulin administration for over a year. Cyclosporine has shown the best results and these can be enhanced by combining it judiciously with other immunosuppressive drugs. However, these drugs are expensive and their long-term administration could lead to major side-effects.

Even though the prospects of preventing type 1 DM are considerably more hopeful than a decade ago, there are formidable challenges. Another decade may pass before we have an acceptable, safe and inexpensive preventive treatment. However, there are rays of hope and we must work on.

LEVELS OF DIABETES PREVENTION

Primary prevention = prevention of diabetes

Ideally, we should aim to prevent the development of new cases of diabetes. It is quite possible though it may not work in every case. The single-point strategy is to identify those at risk (obesity, family history, sedentary lifestyle, faulty diets, etc.) and eliminating those risks through lifestyle alterations.

Ajay, forty-two, is a hardworking executive. However, he is smart enough to realize that good health is imperative for him to excel at his profession. Since both his parents are diabetics, he knows that he has a very high chance of developing it and must prevent it to avoid complications that can cause setbacks in his professional life. Since the day he crossed thirty, he has been undergoing thorough health check-ups every alternate year and has transitioned to a healthy diet. He walks for thirty minutes every day, even when he is on a business tour or a family vacation. He is diabetes-free.

Secondary prevention = prevention of complications of diabetes

This works for those who missed the opportunity to prevent diabetes and sought medical attention after developing it. Aggressive lifestyle alterations along with appropriate medication for diabetes (also blood pressure and cholesterol, if necessary) will help correct blood sugar, blood pressure and blood cholesterol promptly and thus prevent the onset of complications like diabetic retinopathy, diabetic neuropathy, diabetic nephropathy, heart disease and paralytic stroke. For this to be successful, one must diagnose diabetes as early as possible. If you wait till the onset of typical symptoms such as excessive urination, thirst, itching and weight loss, you may lose up to five years between onset and diagnosis. Those five years are critical—do not lose them.

Ahmad, fifty, is a shopkeeper. He is healthy and never had health complaints. Thus he presumed that he did not have any diseases. When his daughter (who has recently started studying medicine) insisted that he go for a routine check-up, he was surprised to discover that he is a diabetic. Luckily, his organ systems did not show any evidence of complications. He was fortunate that his condition was diagnosed early enough. He has resolved to tightly control his lifestyle to maintain quality of life.

Tertiary prevention = prevention of worsening of complications of diabetes

Diabetics who already have some of the above complications when they first visit a specialist need prompt treatment to achieve control over blood sugar, blood pressure, and cholesterol to arrest further deterioration of organ function. Those with mild kidney disease can still prevent the need for dialysis. Those with mild diabetic retinopathy can prevent visual loss. Those with mild heart affection can prevent heart attacks.

Leena, fifty-five, is a devoted homemaker. A year ago, she lost a lot of weight and strength. She postponed medical check-ups till she was finally hospitalized for extreme exhaustion. She was diagnosed with severe diabetes and first stage of diabetic retinopathy. She also had high blood pressure and her electrocardiogram was abnormal. Since then, she is particular about eating healthy food and exercising regularly. She takes her anti-diabetic and blood pressure medications religiously and monitors her blood sugar as well as blood pressure. Her recent health check-up shows that the retinopathy has not worsened and the electrocardiogram has improved. No new complications have developed.

'Superior doctors prevent the disease. Mediocre doctors treat the disease before it is evident. Inferior doctors treat the full-blown disease.'

Ancient Chinese saying, 2600 BC, cited in A.J.M. Boulton, 'The diabetic foot', *Diabetes/Metabolism Research and Reviews* **24**(1): s3–s6.

17

PREGNANCY AND DIABETES

When a diabetic woman gets pregnant, the risk of foetal miscarriage and congenital malformation (birth defects) increases by three to five times compared with a non-diabetic woman. The risk of maternal complications, such as diabetic ketoacidosis, hypertension, hypoglycaemia, and retinopathy is also higher.

There are two different situations in which pregnancy is associated with diabetes: (1) the mother-to-be is a known diabetic or (2) she develops diabetes for the first time during her pregnancy.

The latter type of diabetes is known as gestational diabetes (GD) and it develops due to various hormonal changes and stresses associated with pregnancy in a woman genetically prone to develop the condition. Usually blood glucose levels revert to normal after the delivery but will rise again during subsequent pregnancies. Moreover, these women are more likely to develop type 2 diabetes during the latter part of their lives, particularly if they become overweight.

It is possible to considerably reduce foetal, neonatal and maternal complications associated with pregnancy in diabetic women by strictly controlling blood glucose levels throughout the pregnancy—not only after the diagnosis but right from the stage where conception is planned and attempted. The development of foetal organs is hectic during the six to eight weeks right after the conception. Unfortunately, during this period it is not yet known whether you have successfully conceived and, unless you have pre-planned it methodically, you may not have good control over your blood glucose. Under such circumstances, the risk of abortion as well as birth defects rises considerably. (Since GD usually develops in the third trimester, it is not linked with high risk for congenital malformations.)

If you can control your blood glucose very strictly right from before conception, the complication rates will not be very different from those in a 'normal', non-diabetic pregnancy. If you are committed and get treated by an experienced diabetologist, it is not at all difficult to achieve good blood glucose control. Every 1 per cent reduction in HbA1c during the immediate pre-conception period leads to a 30 per cent reduction in birth defects.

How Can I Minimize the Risk?

If you are a diabetic and would like to conceive, here are some guidelines that you must follow:

1. If you are on diet control alone or insulin therapy, go in for blood glucose and glycosylated haemoglobin tests. If the results indicate good and steady control, go ahead

and conceive. If blood glucose is not controlled, postpone conceiving, start insulin or increase the dose (if already on insulin), achieve control and then conceive.

2. If you are on oral pills, temporarily postpone conceiving, change over to insulin, achieve good and steady control of blood glucose, and then go ahead. Even though it has not been definitely proved that oral anti-diabetics cause birth defects, it is universal convention (except in a few South American countries) to refrain from using oral pills during pregnancy, from before conception.

If you are not a diabetic, stay alert to the possibility of developing GD. To minimize risks associated with GD, you must establish an early diagnosis. Go in for blood glucose tests between the twenty-fourth and twenty-eighth week of your pregnancy; if the results show high values, you should treat it first through diet control and, if needed, with insulin.

If you are at high risk for GD (in cases of GD during previous pregnancy, family history of diabetes, obesity, age above 30 years), you should get your blood glucose tested at the beginning of each trimester. For details on these tests, see Chapter 4.

Poorly controlled GD is associated with a high rate of stillbirth, macrosomia (large-sized foetus), complications during labour and delivery and neonatal hypoglycaemia (immediately after birth). However, birth defects are not as common in babies of GD-afflicted women as in women who were diabetic even before they conceived.

Managing Diabetes during Pregnancy

Generally, the strategies to manage diabetes in pregnant women are the same as those to manage it in normal people. Do take note of the following important points, though:

- During pregnancy, you must absolutely ensure very strict blood glucose control right through. There is nothing to be gained from any carelessness. Your fasting blood glucose should remain between 60 mg% and 95 mg%, while your post-prandial blood glucose should be between 100 mg% and 125 mg%. Also, glycosylated haemoglobin should always be within normal range.

- You must go in for frequent blood glucose estimation to ensure good control. Whether you are a diabetic who got pregnant or a pregnant woman who developed diabetes (GD), you must self-monitor your blood glucose level with capillary blood from a finger prick, at least three times every day. If blood glucose levels are erratic, consult your diabetologist and take prompt corrective measures. Every eight weeks, go for a glycosylated haemoglobin test. If possible, go for a fructosamine test every four weeks.

- During your pregnancy and lactation period, you should consume 500 calories over and above your usual needs to provide for the needs of the growing foetus.

- Immediately after you deliver, your newborn is likely to develop hypoglycaemia. It is vital to test the umbilical blood immediately after delivery and treat hypoglycaemia, if discovered. A neonatologist should be consulted for detailed examination of the baby, not only for hypoglycaemia management but also for diagnosis of birth defects and other complications, if any.

- If you require insulin during pregnancy, use human insulin only. This way, you will not develop antibodies to animal insulin, which could interfere later in life when (and if) you do need insulin to control diabetes.

In the past, diabetes-related complications such as miscarriage and stillbirth, as well as birth defects in the newborn were very common. Gradually, the scenario has changed considerably. Now, diabetic women regularly get pregnant and deliver normal babies. However, compared with non-diabetics, their risks of complications are higher if they are not careful.

CASE STUDY: HOW PRITI PLANNED AND MANAGED HER PREGNANCY

Priti, twenty-eight, is a bit overweight and has a strong family history of diabetes. Three years ago, she delivered a baby girl. In the last two months of her pregnancy, she tested for marginally higher blood glucose values, which she controlled through diet and exercise so that she did not have to take any medications. After the delivery, her blood glucose values reverted to normal. What Priti had was mild gestational diabetes (GD), a type that develops during the last three months of pregnancy and usually disappears soon after delivery.

However, women who develop GD have higher chances of developing permanent type 2 diabetes later in their lives. The very first step Priti took after her delivery was to transition to a prudent lifestyle via diet and exercise. She also made it a point to confirm that her diabetes had indeed disappeared by undergoing a blood glucose test. (In a small percentage of women with GD, blood glucose values do not return to normal after the delivery—they become permanently diabetic.) Since then, she had her blood glucose checked annually to confirm that she did not tilt towards diabetes. Also, Priti actively acquired in-depth knowledge of diabetes and planned her second pregnancy meticulously.

When Priti and her husband, Rahul, decided to have their second child, the first thing Priti did was to go in for temporary family planning; then she monitored her lifestyle and tested her blood glucose, both fasting and post-prandial, along with glycosylated haemoglobin values. She took these steps to confirm that her blood glucose was absolutely normal. She also got assessed for blood pressure, heart and kidney status, and eye health. After getting a green signal from all her doctors, she went ahead to conceive.

Priti knows how important it is to have strict blood glucose control right from conception. The first two weeks in the life of the unborn child are vital: this is the time when the organs develop rapidly. An environment of high blood glucose can prove to be a risk factor and increase chances of birth defects. Priti's decision to first confirm blood glucose control was indeed very wise. She meticulously followed her obstetrician's and diabetologist's advice regarding diet, exercise, medication, and self-monitoring of blood glucose with a glucometer. She did the tests as per the recommended frequency, which increased as her pregnancy advanced into the seventh month. She logged all the values and shared them along with periodic lab-tested blood glucose values with her diabetologist.

Priti also found out that some medications, if consumed in the first trimester, can increase chances of birth defects. Thus, whenever she required any medication, she was careful to take them only after consulting her doctors. She never missed or postponed her appointments with her obstetrician or diabetologist. When they asked her to get a special ultrasound to rule out birth defects, she got it done and was relieved to know that none existed.

Because she took all the precautions, her pregnancy proceeded smoothly. Like in her first pregnancy, there was a small rise in her blood glucose values after major meals. She needed very small doses of insulin, which she learned to self-administer. She was able to maintain fasting and post-prandial blood glucose values below 95 mg% and 125 mg%, respectively. Needless to say, she had a normal delivery. Her newborn weighed normal and did not have any neonatal complications. Priti and Rahul were ecstatic when they heard the child's robust cry.

Priti is keenly aware that her job is not over. Because of her strong family history of type 2 diabetes and her own history of GD, she has a very high chance of developing regular type 2 diabetes later on. She has decided to continue her diet and exercise regimens to prevent excess weight gain. Her blood glucose normalized soon after the second delivery and she does not require insulin any more but she has already marked a date six months down the line on her calendar for her next blood glucose test to ensure that she does not slip into diabetes territory.

18

TREATING DIABETES IN THE 21ST CENTURY

Researchers across the world are working to understand different aspects of diabetes including causes, prevention and management. Every now and then, they make important breakthroughs. It is a continuously evolving process. With the considerable advances made in diabetology over the last decade, prospects for diabetics are getting ever brighter. In the near future, it is likely that immunosuppressant therapy will be perfected, that islet cell transplants will be much more successful, and that there will be implantable miniature artificial pancreas and the wonders of insulin gene therapy. Let us take a look at some of the advances made in diabetes management over the last few decades.

Continuous Glucose Monitoring Systems

In daily use for about a decade now, continuous glucose monitoring systems (CGMS) continuously monitor interstitial fluid glucose, which has a good correlation with blood glucose. Rather than monitor blood glucose, it is easier to monitor interstitial fluid glucose in the abdomen by tucking a disposable sensor into a fat layer just under the skin for seventy-two to ninety-six hours. This sensor continuously monitors tissue fluid glucose and stores a mean glucose value every ten minutes. Real-time versions give a digital display of the level while others store the data retrieved at the end of the monitoring period for a retrospective study. A daily graph based on 144 glucose readings is generated and graphs from three days are superimposed to see variations. The data is also available in pie charts. One gets to know the minimum and maximum values for a given period of twenty-four hours and can study the relationship between variables such as food intake, exercise, anti-diabetic drug administration and their relationship with interstitial fluid glucose. Hypoglycaemia and hyperglycaemia threshold beeps as well as trend arrows are displayed on the screens. A CGMS is a diabetologist's 'Holter monitor'!

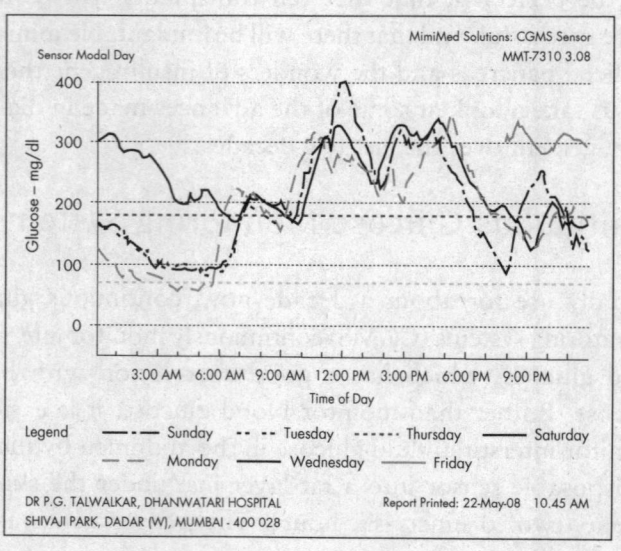

Here is a sample report interpreting the graphs above:

- Shilpa, a long-standing diabetic on pre-mixed insulin three times a day, had poor and brittle blood glucose control. The intra-day fluctuations were documented from as low as below 60 mg% to as high as 400 mg%.
- She was hooked on to a CGMS and her glucose pattern was studied. She has a high post-breakfast peak, a slightly smaller post-lunch peak, a normal post-dinner peak and a tendency to hypoglycaemia in the early morning. The pattern was constant over the three days.
- She should do better with 50:50 pre-mixed insulin during the day and 30:70 pre-mixed insulin around dinner. She would also do better with pre-mixed insulin analogue.

Applications of CGMS

- To study glucose pattern in brittle diabetics (with wide intra-day fluctuations) and those prone to severe hypoglycaemia
- For insulin dose setting in those on insulin pumps
- To study characteristics such as rate of absorption of anti-diabetics to adjust timings for better blood glucose control

HOW SMART IS YOUR PHONE?

The key to better diabetes management may already be in your pocket! Researchers have developed an android-based smartphone with blood glucose estimation capability. The phone has a built-in glucometer, a slot to insert the glucose estimation strip and the provision to store blood glucose data and transmit it to the phone or computer of a third party, such as parents in cases of diabetics who are minors.

Insulin Delivery Systems

Rapid strides have been made in the quality of insulin but insulin delivery systems have lagged behind. Physiologically, insulin is released around the clock in a pulsed manner and delivered directly to the liver via portal circulation. When we inject insulin subcutaneously with syringes or pens, it causes excessive insulin deposits in body parts where it does not have any role to play, while there is low concentration in the liver, the major site of insulin action. Various insulin delivery systems have been designed to overcome this drawback.

Open loop delivery system

In this system, a portable insulin pump can be strapped on to the abdominal wall. (Clinical trials on implantable pumps are under way.) A needle inserted into the subcutaneous tissue on the anterior abdominal wall is attached to the pump via polyethylene tubing. The pump case contains a syringe, the piston of which is driven by the pump. The rate of continuous insulin delivery is adjustable. There is also a provision to give a pre-meal booster dose. With the pump, it is possible to deliver insulin in continuous subcutaneous infusion at a rate mimicking the physiological rate of insulin delivered from the pancreas. For over three decades, many patients, mostly type 1 diabetics, have been using these pumps and it has led to better control of blood glucose level, thus postponing specific complications as compared with conventional insulin administration. Open loop delivery systems have the following limitations, though:

- They administer insulin into the systemic, not portal, circulation.
- There is no sensor to monitor blood/tissue glucose concentrations and a computer to determine dosage.
- Equipment failure may cause too much or too little insulin administration with obvious consequences.
- Cutaneous complications, such as painful lumps and abscesses at the site of needle insertion, have been recorded.
- The pumps are very expensive, the minimum cost being Rs 1 lakh per unit. Even so, many more Indian diabetics have started to use pumps over the last decade.

Case study: Investing in health and career

Sunita, twenty-four, is a brilliant, ambitious young woman. She developed type 1 diabetes at the age of fourteen. She was on multiple insulin injections and always managed her diabetes very efficiently. She completed her management degree from a prestigious university and has been working as a manager in a well-known company. She has learnt a lot about diabetes by reading books, surfing the Web, and attending diabetes education programmes and keeps her blood glucose controlled well. Even so, she recently opted for an insulin pump to continuously deliver insulin around the clock. This way, she need not prick herself several times in a day and chances of hypoglycaemia are minimized. With the new system, she can maintain an even tighter control over her blood glucose levels. She wants to work hard and rise rapidly in her career, and understands the importance of persistent blood glucose control for good health over a long period. That is why she is willing to pay the substantial initial cost of a high-tech insulin pump.

PUMPS THAT CAN PREVENT HYPOGLYCAEMIA

Recently, an upgraded version of conventional insulin pumps has been tested. It is fitted with a built-in sensor to continuously monitor sugar. Like the needle coming out of the pump, the sensors are also tucked into subcutaneous fat over the abdominal wall. The sensors generate substantial data for precise adjustment of anti-diabetic medications. Stand-alone sensors have been in use for about a decade while combined insulin pumps with sensors have been available for routine use for around two years now. Insulin pumps with automatic low glucose suspension of insulin delivery are the latest advance in this field. When sugar level dips below a preset level, which is adjustable, the pump automatically suspends insulin delivery for two hours. This safety feature pre-empts episodes of severe hypoglycaemia, especially at night.

Closed loop delivery system

A closed loop delivery system is one in which there is a built-in sensor to monitor prevailing glucose concentration in the interstitial fluid, a computer to analyse the data generated by the sensor and to decide insulin dosage, and a pump to deliver the insulin—all working in an integrated manner. Two examples of such a system are biostators and implantable artificial pancreases. A biostator contains the glucose sensor, computer, pump and a printer to automatically record all biochemical data. However, such an artificial pancreas is bulky and can be used only in hospital or research laboratory settings. It is hardly used in clinical practice now. Meanwhile, considerable progress has been made in developing an implantable artificial pancreas, which is a miniaturized pancreas that can be implanted in the abdominal cavity. Of the three vital components of an artificial pancreas, two—miniature matchbox-sized pump and microcomputer—have been developed, while research is under way to develop a sensitive, reliable and durable mini sensor. The completion and use of miniature implantable artificial pancreases would be a major breakthrough in diabetes management.

BREAKTHROUGH IN OPERATIONALIZING ARTIFICIAL PANCREASES

While the development of implantable artificial pancreases is progressing gradually, external artificial pancreases with wireless linking of the three vital components positioned outside the body (sensor, pump, computer) has become operational.

Recently, eighteen adolescents aged between fifteen and eighteen years were successfully hooked on to artificial pancreases in a camp setting in Israel. Off-the-shelf sensors were used to continuously monitor their glucose concentration while insulin pumps continuously delivered the required amount of insulin. Both the sensor and the pump were looped wirelessly with a laptop computer loaded with software to receive inputs from sensors, analyse the data, decide on the insulin requirement and send outputs to the pumps to deliver insulin as required. All this while, the patients could move freely and participate in camp activities.

During the period that these adolescents were hooked on to artificial pancreases, their blood glucose levels were very steady; both high sugar peaks as well as low sugar dips were avoided. The entire process was automated; there was no need for manual blood glucose estimation or decisions on insulin dosage and physical administration. Diabetologists and software engineers closely monitored vital clinical data and the patients. This success of artificial pancreases in a non-hospital set-up is a major milestone and will pave the way for regular use outside hospitals.

Pancreatic Transplantation

The first successful pancreas transplant (actually part of a simultaneous kidney-pancreas transplant) was done in 1966 by Dr William Kelly and Dr Richard Lillehei at the University of Minnesota, Minneapolis, USA. Since then, pancreatic transplants have become increasing acceptable. In most cases, the pancreas comes from cadaver donors, though, theoretically, a living person can donate a part of his or her pancreas.

This is the most natural approach to maintain euglycaemia (normal blood glucose level) in diabetics. Insulin secretion from successfully transplanted pancreas occurs in a need-based manner and automatically stops in a fasting state. This means that hypoglycaemia is naturally prevented, as it would be in a non-diabetic. However, there are several immunological and technical problems in the process, which is why the surgery can be done only at a few highly specialized centres. The problems are being resolved gradually and the success rate of pancreatic transplantation is looking up, though it is much lower than that of kidney transplantation.

In patients with diabetic nephropathy and end-stage renal failure, doctors perform simultaneous pancreas and kidney transplants. In fact, pancreas is transplanted only in those patients who also need kidney transplants, as both cases necessitate lifelong immunosuppressant therapy. The use of cyclosporine as an immunosuppressant has considerably reduced graft rejection rates compared with azathioprine.

More than fifty institutions in the West perform pancreas transplants and the mean one-year survival rate of grafts is gradually improving. The maximum experience has been developed by the pancreatic transplantation team of the University of Minnesota Medical School.

Islet Cells Transplantation

This has been successful in experiments on animals and, in a limited manner, in the case of human diabetics. Tremendous research is currently under way to improve the success rate of islet cell transplantation techniques for human use. Two potential advantages of this technique are that (1) it is a much simpler procedure for recipients than pancreatic transplantation and (2) in vitro manipulations can be performed on islet cells before a transplant to reduce immunogenicity (chance of rejection by the host).

Other Directions in Insulin Research

Insulin analogues

Recombinant DNA technology is being used to produce several insulin analogues via biological engineering. These analogues have the same biological activity as human insulin but have different absorption patterns to suit the needs of diabetics. Certain analogues are absorbed faster than human insulin and can be used in those whose post-prandial blood glucose is difficult to control and those who are prone to late post-prandial hypoglycaemia. Other analogues remain in circulation longer than intermediate-acting human insulin and hence are more suitable for patients who have difficulty in controlling fasting hyperglycaemia and are prone to hypoglycaemia, particularly late at night and early in the morning.

In insulin analogues, certain amino acids of insulin polypeptide chains (not involved in the stability and biological activity of insulin) are substituted to create analogues with more desirable action profiles. Rapid-acting analogues (insulin lispro [Humalog], insulin glulisine [Apidra], insulin aspart [NovoRapid]) and long-acting analogues (insulin glargine [Lantus], insulin detemir [Levemir]) are already available, while more are being clinically tested. Degludec, a long-acting insulin analogue meant to be injected twice a week is in an advanced stage of development, as is a rapid-acting insulin analogue which gets absorbed even faster than others in its class. It is ideal for post-prandial glucose control and preventing late post-prandial hypoglycaemia.

Alternative routes to administer insulin

What with the limitations of administering insulin subcutaneously, medical researchers are continuously exploring the options of peritoneal infusion. To an extent, this route mimics the normal pattern of insulin circulation. Implantable intra-abdominal devices administer insulin but obstruction of an implantable catheter can pose a major complication.

Inhalation route

Strips containing dry powered insulin are introduced into a device that releases insulin when the patient inhales. The insulin gets absorbed into the lung's blood circulation. Exubera, the first such 'inhaled' insulin, was introduced in the west some years ago but soon withdrawn, probably because it did not do well commercially and also because there was a possibility that the aerosol suspending agent was carcinogenic. The lung route has not been totally abandoned though. Research on safer aerosols and better devices is under way.

Buccal route

Insulin in aerosol form is sprayed over the buccal mucosa, through which it is absorbed into the circulation. The only country where this product is available is Ecuador (South America).

Nasal route

Intranasal administration of insulin has been used experimentally for several years. A major problem is that the adjuvants[1] used to facilitate trans-nasal absorption of insulin cause nasal irritation. Moreover, there are no large-scale trials to study variations in insulin absorption in the case of a diabetic with a diseased nasal mucosa.

Oral insulin

Since the insulin molecule is a protein, it is split into its constituent amino acids by the enzymes in the upper gastrointestinal tract before it can be absorbed into the bloodstream. Thus it is totally ineffective when administered orally. However, considering that most patients resist injecting insulin, several researchers are attempting to develop an envelope or coating, which would prevent digestion of insulin and allow its absorption intact. Biocon, an Indian biotechnology and pharmaceutical company, is at the forefront of the development of oral insulin.

Insulin gene therapy

This is an exciting new subject, which has opened up the possibility of the impossible: a cure for diabetes. Since diabetes involves defects in many genes, there are many ways in which genes can be used to treat and prevent it. It has been demonstrated that a human insulin gene can be introduced into cells that originally did not synthesize insulin and that

---

1 An adjuvant is a pharmacological/immunological agent that modifies the effect of a drug by playing a supportive role. They are often included in vaccines to enhance the recipient's immune response to a supplied antigen while minimizing injected foreign material.

these cells can be introduced into animals where they can function in a predictable and physiological manner—they can secrete insulin as per demand and shut down insulin synthesis when blood glucose approaches basal normal range.

Another approach is to use the gene that determines tissue sensitivity to insulin. Mutation of the SHIP2 gene is associated with severe reduction in tissue sensitivity to insulin, leading to diabetes. If this is tackled, insulin sensitivity can be increased and blood glucose normalized. Yet another approach is to use the gene that will prevent overgrowth of blood vessels in the retina, which causes diabetic retinopathy leading to blindness. Though there are several challenges to be overcome before gene therapy in diabetes becomes a reality, it is encouraging that the possibility exists.

Development of Immunosuppressants

A growing body of evidence suggests that type 1 diabetes is caused by auto-immune destruction of insulin-producing beta cells of the pancreas. Auto-antibodies against insulin, beta cell surfaces, and islet cells cytoplasm are often present in some newly diagnosed type 1 diabetics. Recent therapeutic efforts have been focused on immunosuppressive agents to counter this. Initial attempts to use steroids, antilymphocytic serum, azathioprine, and plasmaphersis have been inconclusive but recent pilot trials in 40 type 1 diabetics using cyclosporine have been encouraging. These trials demonstrated that early treatment with cyclosporine can induce remission from insulin dependence (self-destruction of beta cells in the pancreas is halted and the cells start producing insulin); as many as half the patients do not require insulin after a year.

Embryonic stem cell research

Cells from an embryo freshly fertilized via in vitro fertilization can be grown in a laboratory and selective growth and differentiation of pancreatic beta cells can be promoted. Research on various aspects of this highly potential area is under way. When successful, it will offer an exciting alternative to pancreatic and islet cell transplantation.

Emerging Anti-diabetic Agents (Other Than Insulin)

Over the last decade, several new agents that act very differently as compared with established agents (metformin, sulphonylureas, glinides, alpha glucosidase inhibitors) have joined the armamentarium of anti-diabetic medications. In spite of these new agents, only a few diabetics can attain glycaemic goals, all because of the progressive nature of type 2 diabetes. Thus, the relentless search for new classes of anti-diabetics continues. Here is an overview of some new agents that have emerged on the horizon:

Colesevelam hydrochloride

This bile acid sequestrant is primarily used to treat high cholesterol conditions. Recent clinical trials have shown that this compound can also significantly lower blood glucose.

Pramlintide

While insulin has been the mainstay of diabetes therapy, the quest for better control with fewer unwanted side effects (weight gain, hypoglycaemia) and freedom from constant dosage adjustment has fuelled the search for newer agents. Anti-diabetic therapy is continuously evolving.

We know that diabetes is a disease with multiple hormonal defects. Besides insulin deficiency, there is also a deficiency of amylin, which beta cells secrete with insulin. The natural actions of amylin complement those of insulin; amylin reduces appetite, delays gastric emptying, and suppresses inappropriate post-prandial rise of glucagon, thus suppressing glucose production in the liver. Pramlintide, a synthetic analogue of amylin, is injected subcutaneously twice a day. It has been available in the USA since 2005 and is indicated as an adjuvant to insulin in type 1 and type 2 diabetics who fail to reach their glycaemic targets.

The pros of pramlintide are weight reduction, relative freedom from hypoglycaemia, and a simple dosage schedule that obviates dosage titration. Side effects include nausea, occasional vomiting, and hypoglycaemia due to insulin, which is co-administered. While gastrointestinal side effects reduce over time, hypoglycaemia can be tackled by reducing insulin dosage.

Sergiflozin and dapagiflozin

These agents reduce blood glucose level by blocking reabsorption of glucose by the kidneys. This is a novel approach as the action is not dependent on beta cells, insulin resistance, or type of diabetes. Initial trials have confirmed efficacy and safety.

Advances in Treating Diabetic Complications

Diabetic nephropathy

The importance of meticulous blood glucose control in preventing nephropathy has been established. Moreover, it is now possible to catch the onset of diabetic nephropathy earlier via various tests to detect microalbuminuria. We know that hypertension accelerates the progression of nephropathy and should be aggressively treated. There are numerous anti-hypertensive agents (with different mechanisms of action) to choose from, depending on individual contexts. Angiotensin converting enzyme (ACE) inhibitors and angiotensin receptor blockers (ARBs) reduce microalbuminuria and are very useful in treating hypertension in diabetics. They also slow down the deterioration rate from early nephropathy to end-stage renal failure. They can be started at high normal (towards higher limit of normal) blood pressure level in those who have microalbuminuria. Of course, it is evident that those who have diabetic nephropathy must transition to a low-protein diet. Orally active agent ruboxistaurin has shown promise in managing diabetic nephropathy. It works by inhibiting the protein kinase C enzyme, which plays a central role in damaging the inner layer (endothelium) of small blood vessels, particularly in the retina, kidneys and nerves.

Diabetic retinopathy

ACE inhibitors, particularly ramipril and lisinopril, help prevent diabetic retinopathy and can be given even to diabetics with normal blood pressure. Retinal photocoagulation[2] using an argon ion laser can prevent blindness in those with proliferative diabetic retinopathy and maculopathy but it is essentially a preventive measure and not useful in patients with severe visual impairment. Laser is also used to perform vitrectomy[3] in diabetics in whom vitreous haemorrhage does not get absorbed within twelve weeks. This guards against future retinal detachment. Orally active agent ruboxistaurin has shown promise in managing diabetic retinopathy as well.

Other Emerging Solutions

Bariatric surgery: This is a new direction of solutions for morbidly obese type 2 diabetics. Among its various surgical procedures, gastric bypass with pancreaticobiliary diversion and gastric banding are more effective. Bariatric surgery

---

2 Retinal photocoagulation is a process in which a laser beam is directed on to a leaking retinal capillary to permanently seal the leak.
3 Vitrectomy is a surgical procedure to remove unhealthy tissue and fluids from the eye. It is done in cases of retinal detachment to improve surgical access to the retina and also when there is blood inside the eye and is not getting cleared naturally.

causes malabsorption of food (some of the ingested food is not assimilated but is passed out via faeces) and reduced food intake due to a feeling of fullness in the abdomen. Patients undergoing gastric bypass surgery lose, on average, 40 per cent of their weight. All of them show significant improvements in blood glucose control. In fact, in 82 per cent cases, anti-diabetic medications are not required any longer for blood glucose control because bariatric surgery increases the levels of incretin hormones, which increase insulin secretion, which makes anti-diabetics redundant. Several obese diabetics now opt for the surgical approach to tackle their dual problem of obesity and diabetes.

Anti-diabetic vaccines

Several scientists are working to develop molecules that will prevent beta cell destruction by auto-antibodies in recently diagnosed type 1 diabetics and halt the progression of diabetes. Israeli scientists are at the forefront of this exciting research frontier.

Appendix I

TAKING CARE OF YOUR FEET

Diabetics, especially those who have had the condition for a long time and/or are poorly controlled, have a very high risk of developing an array of foot complications such as infections, non-healing ulcers, and gangrene. They are more vulnerable than non-diabetics because they have poor blood supply in the lower limbs owing to atherosclerotic peripheral vascular disease; they have impaired sensation in the legs and feet owing to diabetic peripheral neuropathy; and they have an increased susceptibility to infection. To avoid these complications, diabetics should take meticulous care of their feet, even as he manages his overall diabetic condition energetically.

If a diabetic neglects his feet, complications gradually set in and may ultimately result in gangrene, in which case the affected foot may have to be amputated. A diabetic is seventeen times more likely to get gangrene in the lower limbs, compared with a non-diabetic.

Foot Care Regimen
- Wash your feet at least twice a day with mild soap and lukewarm (never hot) water.
- Dry your feet gently with a soft towel, taking care to remove all the excess moisture between the toes.

- If your skin is dry, rub in a mild lubricant such as coconut oil, petroleum jelly or cold cream every night before you turn in.
- Trim your toenails regularly. Always cut straight across, never close to the skin. Make sure there are no jagged edges.
- Inspect your feet every day for any cuts, blisters, boils, or wounds. If you find any, consult a doctor and treat the area promptly.
- Never walk barefoot, not even at home.
- Never use a hot-water bottle on your feet, as your local sensation might be impaired and you might end up burning your feet.
- To protect your toes, wear broad soft canvas or leather shoes. Avoid open-toed chappals, sandals and footwear made of rubber or plastic. Inspect the insoles of shoes daily for any small stones, nails, etc.
- Break in new shoes gradually by wearing them for a short time only, to start with. Always buy shoes in the evening when your foot size is at its maximum.
- Wear cotton socks, preferably seamless ones. Avoid socks with very tight elasticated bands, for these will hamper blood circulation to your legs.
- Do not cut any corns or calluses yourself. Always consult a doctor.
- Do not apply any strong chemicals to your feet.
- Avoid tobacco in any form.
- Exercise regularly to boost blood circulation.

Appendix II

PREVENTING GUM AND TOOTH DISEASES

Diabetics, especially those who have poor blood glucose control, are highly vulnerable to diseases of the gums and the teeth.

Diseases of the Gums

Diabetics have reduced capacity to fight infections, particularly when blood glucose is high. What is more, associated salivary gland affection and dehydration cause dryness in the oral cavity. These conditions make diabetics vulnerable to diseases of the gums and teeth.

In the initial stage, the gums show mild swelling and become spongy. If blood glucose remains persistently high, gums get infected with bacteria. As the swelling increases due to pus formation, a foul smell emanates and the gums start to bleed. If the process is unchecked, the jaw bones suffer wear and tear, leading to teeth sockets getting loosened and teeth tending to fall. In diabetics who consume tobacco, deterioration of gum condition is much faster. Severe gum infection places extra stress on the body, which causes deterioration in blood glucose control, which further aggravates gum infection . . . And thus a vicious cycle sets in.

Diseases of the Oral Cavity

When blood glucose is very high (for instance, fasting level over 250 mg%), there is excessive urination and that dehydrates the body, a symptom of which is a very dry mouth. In uncontrolled diabetics, this problem is aggravated because the salivary glands malfunction and form lesser saliva than normal. This usually leads to dental caries.

Uncontrolled diabetics are also exposed to fungal infection of the oral cavity by *Candida albicans* (candidiasis or thrush). The affected patient develops whitish patches on the tongue, tonsillar area, buccal mucous membrane, and throat and food pipe. He will also have a sore mouth, pain in the tonsillar area, and difficulty swallowing. Uncontrolled diabetics who use artificial dentures suffer from painful ulcers in the oral cavity and on the tongue. They develop oral herpes simplex viral infection as well as lichen planus more frequently than non-diabetics.

Preventive Measures

- Maintain your blood glucose persistently. With prudent diet control, regular exercise, and regimented anti-diabetic medications, it is not difficult to attain your blood glucose goals. As a diabetic, you have no other alternative.
- Avoid tobacco and tobacco products as well as *paan*, *supari*, *gutkha*, and so on.
- Brush your teeth at least twice a day.
- Visit a dental surgeon every six months for a routine proactive check-up and ultrasonic scaling of gums, if required.

Appendix III

MIXING INSULIN

1. 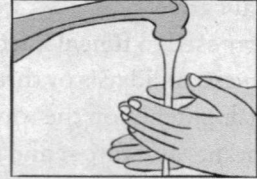 First of all, wash your hands thoroughly. Cleanliness prevents infections.

2. 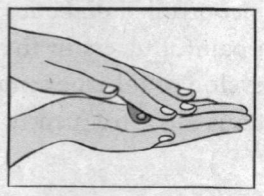 Slowly roll the vial of cloudy (NPH, Huminsulin-N) insulin between your hands. Do not shake it. Make sure that the cloudy insulin is mixed completely and that there are no insulin crystals left at the bottom of the vial.

3. 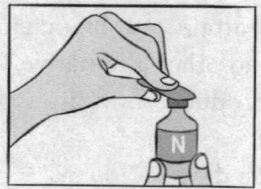 Clean the rubber stopper of each vial with a spirit swab. In this example, we are going to draw a total of 30 units of insulin: 20 units of cloudy insulin and 10 units of regular (crystalline/plain) insulin (Huminsulin-R, Actrapid).

4. 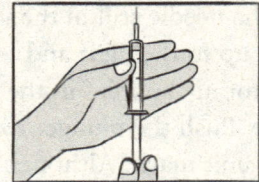 First, draw air into the syringe up to the dose of cloudy insulin. In this example, it is 20 units. So, draw air up to the 20-unit mark.

5. 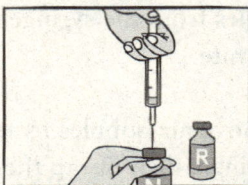 Insert the needle through the stopper of the vial of cloudy insulin and push the 20 units of air into the vial. Keep the vial upright and remove the syringe. Do not draw any of the cloudy insulin yet.

6. 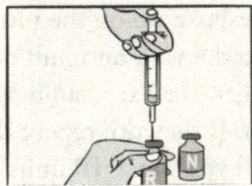 Now, fill the syringe with air equal to the number of units of clear insulin. In this example, it is 10 units.

7. 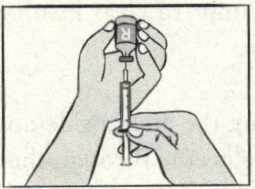 Leave the needle stuck in the vial. Turn the vial upside down. Pull the plunger down to draw 15 units of clear insulin, 5 units more than the 10 units we are using for this example.

8.

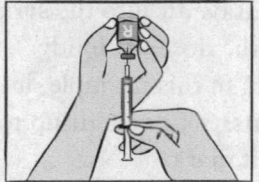

With the needle still in the vial, hold it up to the light and check for air bubbles in the syringe. Push the plunger to the 10-unit mark. Although this air is not dangerous if injected, you should remove any bubbles from the syringe so that your insulin dose is accurate.

9.

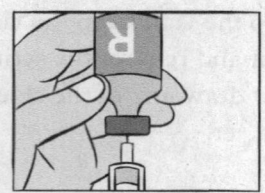

To remove air bubbles from the syringe, flick or tap the syringe at the site of the bubbles. This will push the bubbles to the top of the syringe. Push up on the plunger to force the bubbles back into the vial, and pull down on the plunger to draw 10 units of clear insulin again. No air bubbles should appear. If they do, repeat the flicking and pushing step until you draw 10 units of clear insulin without any bubbles. Then, remove the needle from the vial with 10 units of clear insulin in the syringe.

10.

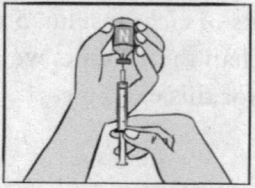

Holding the vial upside down, put the needle through the stopper of the cloudy insulin vial. You need 20 units of cloudy insulin for this example. Since you already have 10

units of clear insulin in the syringe, pull the plunger out to the 30-unit mark, the total of two types of insulin. Remove the needle from the vial.

11. 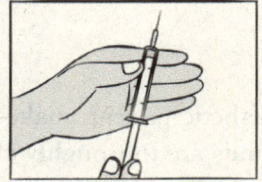 Check again for bubbles. Rarely will you find them at this step but if you do, discard this syringe and start again from Step 1.

Appendix IV

INJECTING INSULIN

Before injecting yourself or the diabetic patient, make sure that the injection site and your hands are thoroughly clean. Use spirit or eau de Cologne to clean the skin.

1. 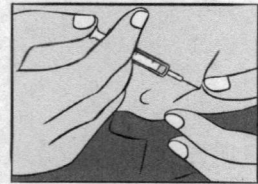 With one hand, grip the syringe. With the other, pinch up some skin.

2. 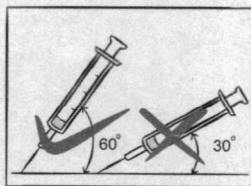 Hold the syringe at an angle of 60° to the spot where you want to inject.

3. 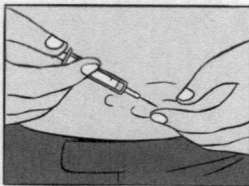 Press the skin gently with the needle so that it 'dimples'.

4. 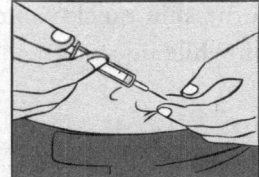 Insert the needle to its full length.

5. 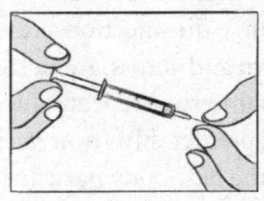 Let go the skin and grasp the lower end of the syringe. With the other hand gently raise the plunger little away. If blood appears in the syringe, withdraw the needle and start again about 1 inch away from the spot. If no blood appears, place your thumb on top of the plunger and inject insulin. Quickly withdraw the needle and press firmly over the injection site with a clean, dry cotton swab for a few seconds. Do not rub.

Tips to Inject Insulin Virtually Painlessly

- If you refrigerate your insulin vials and pens, take them out of the refrigerator and keep them at room temperature for five to ten minutes before injecting. Insulin must be injected at ambient temperature.
- Do not inject insulin immediately after applying spirit/ alcohol to the spot. Wait for two minutes to let it dry.
- Always use an insulin syringe with no. 32 needle.
- If you can afford it, use an insulin pen instead of a syringe.

- While injecting, pierce through the skin quickly and do not change the needle's direction while injecting.

Ideal Spot to Inject Insulin

The best spot for injection is one where a loose fold of flesh can be pinched up. You should change the injection site every day, moving about 1 inch up or down and across. An unsightly lump will develop if you use the same spot repeatedly. Also insulin is absorbed slower and unpredictably from such an area. The following figure depicts the best body parts (circled areas) for insulin injections.

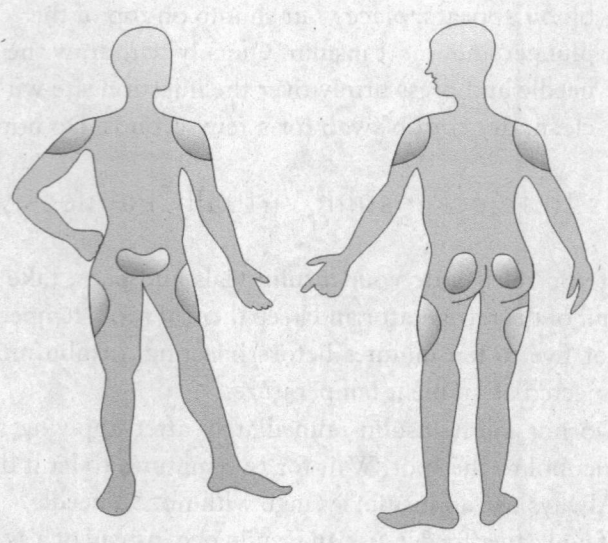

Appendix V

USING INSULIN PENS
(REUSABLES AND DISPOSABLES)

1. 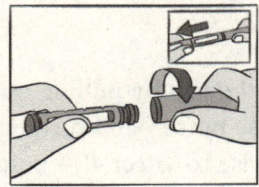 Pull off the pen cap. Unscrew the pen apart.

2. 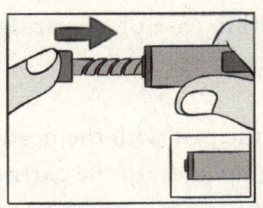 Press in the head of the piston rod as far as it goes.

3. 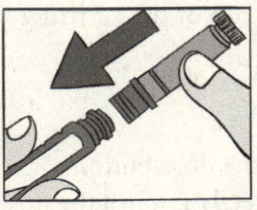 Insert the insulin cartridge into the cartridge holder. The colour-coded cap end goes in first.

4. 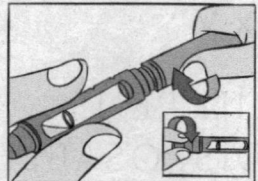 Screw the two parts of the insulin pen tightly together till you hear a click. Then, screw on the insulin needle. Remember, before inserting the cartridge of cloudy insulin (Mixtard, Novomix), roll it in your palms for about 20 seconds or 20 times.

5. 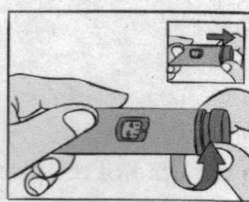 Prime the pen by pulling out the dose button and turning it clockwise to select 4 (4 units) in case of a new cartridge or 1 (1 unit) in case of a cartridge already in use.

6. 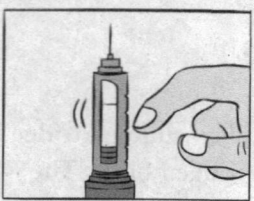 Hold the pen with the needle facing up and tap the cartridge holder to raise any air bubbles to the top of the cartridge.

7. 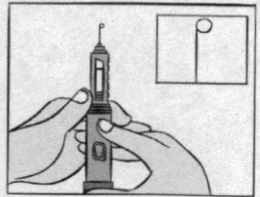 Press the dose button completely in until the dose display window shows zero. Confirm that a drop of insulin has appeared at the tip of the needle. This means that the pen

is primed and ready for use. If a drop of insulin does not appear at the needle tip, repeat steps 5–7 till it does.

8. 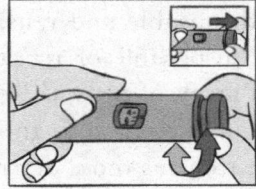 To select the dose, pull out the dose button and rotate it clockwise till you get to the required dose.

9. 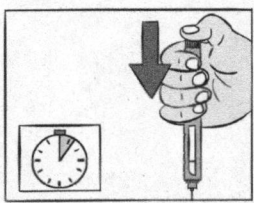 The actual injecting procedure and sites are the same for syringes and pens. To inject insulin via a pen, press the dose button completely till the display shows zero and you hear or feel a click. Then, leave the needle under the skin for about 10 seconds. Withdraw the needle and replace the needle cap followed by the pen cap. While insulin manufacturers do recommend that you change the needle after each injection, if you want to economize and if you ensure proper hygiene, you can use the same needle up to ten times.

The procedure to inject insulin from a disposable syringe is essentially the same as that for a reusable syringe. Since disposables are available in ready-to-use form with the insulin cartridge inserted by the manufacturer, you can bypass the first four steps. The advantage of a disposable insulin syringe has to be traded off against the higher cost of insulin per unit.

Note: Several insulin brands are available in the market. Some offer both types of pens (disposable and reusable) while others have only one type (disposable or reusable). With each brand offering its own array of pens, the exact operating procedure may differ from one brand to another, though the basic principles are the same as those described here. Just follow the use instructions on the package if you face any problems.

Appendix VI

PREPARING FOR MEDICAL CONSULTATIONS

I. Choosing Your Doctor

You will need to approach one or more of the following doctors for your diabetes-related health-care needs.

Family physician

He will help you with your day-to-day problems, arranging health check-ups, and choosing a specialist. Even if you have directly approached a consultant for diabetes management, you should always keep your family physician posted about your health status with reference to diabetes; he is trained to manage diabetes in a broad, generalized manner. In fact, in rural and semi-urban areas where specialists are not easily available, family physicians regularly treat diabetics.

Consultant physician

He is a doctor of medicine (MD) in a broad specialty known as internal or general medicine; diabetes is included in his field of activity as a consultant. He is qualified to prevent, diagnose, and treat various complications of diabetes in the early stages. Most general physicians are affiliated to hospitals where they can arrange for their patients to be treated, if need arises. Many suffix the term 'diabetologist' to their names though most do not practise diabetology exclusively. Having said that, in case a diabetologist or endocrinologist is not available, it is a consultant general physician who can take decisions regarding insulin initiation, major changes in insulin dosage and treating complications and emergencies in diabetics, even those with severe diabetes. In fact, some general physicians with experience, aptitude and knowledge can treat almost any diabetic.

Endocrinologist and diabetologist

An endocrinologist is a specialist in diseases of the endocrine system. He is an MD in endocrinology, having studied it for two years after completing his MD in general medicine. Besides diabetes, he treats diseases of the thyroid, adrenal, pituitary, and other endocrine glands. A diabetologist is usually a consultant physician who devotes all his professional time to treating diabetes and accumulates solid experience in preventing and managing diabetes and its complications. Few universities offer a postgraduate degree exclusively in diabetology (in India, the University of Madras is the only one) so most diabetologists gain experience and recognition by working in departments in large hospitals, including teaching hospitals, and dealing exclusively with diabetics. Some universities and institutions offer diploma/certificate courses, ranging from a few weeks to two years, for qualified doctors. Doctors who undergo these courses also practise as diabetologists; several acquire good experience and expertise in controlling blood glucose levels, though they lack a strong foundation in general medicine. Diabetologists and endocrinologists are experts at controlling blood glucose levels as well as preventing, diagnosing and managing various complications of diabetes. Many patients seek direct consultations with them.

Ophthalmologist

This in an eye specialist. Every type 2 diabetic should consult an ophthalmologist (not, mind you, an optometrist in a spectacles shop) soon after diagnosis of diabetes, and every type 1 diabetic should see him five years after diagnosis. Thereafter, as long as the eyes are not affected by diabetes, one should go for yearly eye tests by a general ophthalmologist. A patient who has diabetic retinopathy and needs laser photocoagulation to arrest deterioration should consult an ophthalmologist experienced in laser therapy and equipped to deliver it. Diabetics with advanced/complicated diabetic retinopathy and those with retinal detachment should go to a retina specialist, who is experienced at carrying out relevant surgical interventions.

Nephrologist

This is a kidney specialist, a 'medical' kidney specialist in fact, different from a urologist, who specializes in surgical aspects of the urinary tract including kidneys. Usually, diabetologists tackle the prevention and diagnosis of kidney disease and the prevention of its progression in diabetics. A nephrologist is consulted in cases with advanced kidney disease and where additional diseases responsible for kidney dysfunction are associated.

Other specialists

Among those commonly called upon for joint consultation are cardiologists and cardiac surgeons, foot surgeons, peripheral vascular surgeons, plastic surgeons and interventional radiologists. Depending on the complications in an individual patient, a decision is taken by the patient's primary doctor (usually a diabetologist) in consultation with the patient and his family. While treating your blood glucose, your diabetes specialist constantly thinks about all the organs likely to be affected by diabetes. Periodically, he also orders appropriate tests to assess your organ systems and give you preventive/ therapeutic medicines to prevent and treat associated complications. When complications reach a certain level, a system specialist's help is sought. Diabetologists work closely with various specialists for the patient's benefit.

CASE STUDY: WHEN SPECIALISTS WORK TOGETHER TOWARDS SUCCESS

Gopal is sixty years old and has been a diabetic for seven years. He used to be a heavy smoker till five years ago, and still smokes a couple of cigarettes every day. Two years ago, he started experiencing pain in his right calf while walking. His diabetologist explained to him that this was due to a complication of diabetes known as peripheral vascular disease. In this condition, the internal diameter of arteries supplying blood to his thighs, legs, and feet is irregular and narrowed, thus reducing blood supply. In resting condition, the calf receives just about adequate blood supply but the increased demand (while walking) is not met, causing calf pain. The diabetologist added that diabetics are more prone to peripheral vascular disease and, in Gopal's case, additional risk factors were smoking, high LDL cholesterol and high blood pressure. Besides pills to control blood glucose, Gopal was prescribed atorvastatin tablets to control his LDL cholesterol, telmisartan tablets to prevent high blood pressure, and aspirin tablets as blood thinners so that he could have smoother blood circulation, particularly in his lower limbs. He was repeatedly advised to shun smoking completely.

Recently, Gopal injured the big toe on his right foot. Due to negligence, the injured area got infected and he developed an abscess. His diabetologist found that besides the abscess, he also had significantly impaired blood supply to the right foot. His suspicion was supported by an arterial Doppler test. He consulted an interventional radiologist, who did a right lower limb angiography to confirm and delineate the area of narrowing in the right leg artery. He then performed an angioplasty to open up the narrowed artery and inserted a stent to maintain its patency (unobstructed openness) over a long term. Angioplasty and stenting together improved blood supply to Gopal's foot.

Subsequently, a foot surgeon was consulted. He made a wide incision and drained out all the accumulated pus and removed all the dead tissue. Since the interventional radiologist's interventions had significantly improved blood supply to the right foot, the wound started to heal rapidly. When all dead tissue was separated and underlying tissue was healthy, a plastic surgeon performed a skin graft to close the wound early. If left unattended, it would have taken three months for the wound to heal completely and there was always the risk of recurring infection.

Gopal's diabetologist worked closely with an interventional radiologist, a foot surgeon and a plastic surgeon and thus helped Gopal avoid a likely toe amputation. Now, Gopal has quit tobacco totally and is relearning the importance of tight and persistent blood glucose control along with control of blood pressure and cholesterol levels.

II. Fix an Appointment

Always fix an appointment. Do not force the doctor to see you out of turn or to give you an early, out of turn appointment unless there is an emergency. Common requests such as 'Please see me today,' 'I am ready to wait for long hours,' 'You can see me after your last patient,' 'It is ok with me even if you take me in at 10 p.m.' are very unfair on the doctor who has been working very hard since early morning. The quality of consultation is also likely to suffer during forced consultations. Please avoid calling the doctor's personal cell number for appointments: doctors do not personally maintain appointment diaries; they are concentrating all the time on patient examination. Their cell phone is meant for emergencies and for their assistants to communicate with them. Therefore, call the landline number at the doctor's clinic for an appointment.

III. Carry All Relevant Documents

1. If you have a current prescription, please carry it. If you do not, carry the list of your medicines with exact doses. In fact, it is better to carry all the prescribed medicines. In case you are not taking all the medicines prescribed to you or are taking them in different doses, you must bring this to the doctor's attention during the consultation. If you don't, your doctor is likely to assume that you comply fully with your prescription and will adjust your anti-diabetic medications accordingly. This can cause complications, so be clear and honest.

CASE STUDIES: NEVER WITHHOLD INFORMATION FROM YOUR DOCTOR

Rajesh decided to consult a diabetologist as his blood glucose level was very high despite taking insulin and medicines prescribed by a physician. He shared his current prescription and latest blood glucose report (fasting 232 mg%; post-prandial 405 mg%) with the diabetologist but did not disclose that he had discontinued the afternoon dose of insulin and reduced the evening dose from 20 units to 10 units. He also refrained from mentioning that he had relaxed his diet and exercise regimens! The diabetologist assumed that Rajesh was taking insulin as prescribed, and escalated his dose, because his blood glucose was still high. Rajesh went off and started taking insulin as per the new prescription. He also focused on his diet and exercise, which he had ignored for some time. Within a couple of days, his blood glucose dropped to a dangerously low level. Had he disclosed the actual insulin dose he was taking at the time of consultation, the diabetologist would not have increased his dosage; instead, he would have advised him to start taking insulin exactly as per the prescribed dose and get back after one week with a fresh blood glucose report. He would have adjusted the insulin dose only after verifying the fresh report and thus the low blood glucose reaction would have been averted.

Another common mistake patients make is to avoid mentioning that they missed the insulin dose just prior to blood glucose testing. In such cases, the blood glucose report is likely to be misinterpreted. Shanta is on insulin twice a day, before breakfast and before dinner. Despite repeated advice from her doctor about learning how to self-inject, she depends on a nurse who stays in the neighbourhood. Once in a while, the nurse is unable to come over and Shanta misses her insulin shot. Recently, Shanta's fasting blood glucose level was 254 mg% and her post-lunch blood glucose level was 165 mg%. Now, Shanta's doctor was very alert and sharp. Even though a diabetic can have higher fasting blood glucose than post-prandial, he decided to verify whether Shanta had missed the previous evening's dose before increasing her insulin dosage. The cat was out of the bag! If the doctor had assumed that Shanta took insulin as per his advice on all days, including on and before the day of the blood test, he would have unnecessarily increased her evening dose, causing a low blood glucose reaction in the middle of the night.

Disclose everything to your doctor. Do not hide any medical information. The doctor has pledged to keep all information confidential.

2. Carry all laboratory reports and reports of other investigations (such as X-rays, ultrasounds, electrocardiograms) arranged chronologically.
3. If you have been hospitalized in the past, carry the discharge card.

IV. Make the Most of the Meeting

Before you meet the doctor, carefully think about all the complaints you have and all the other aspects of your health that bother you. Make a shortlist so that you don't forget to discuss any important matter. Articulate your complaints well. Mention the most troublesome symptoms first but do not omit even the slightest symptoms.

ACKNOWLEDGEMENTS

I would like to thank my patients who have patiently listened to me and given me an opportunity to hone my skills of patient education and to learn about their exact requirements as regards the contents and presentation formats of educational material. I would also like to express my gratitude to Ms Soly James, Chief Dietician, S.L. Raheja Hospital, Mumbai. I would also like to thank my commissioning editor, Mudita Chauhan-Mubayi, and all her colleagues at Penguin Books for expertly editing my manuscript and producing this book.